PRAISE FOR *KNOW YOUR ENDO*

"Just the right blend of empathy, insight, and practical advice. Murnane has created an excellent guide to self-care."

—KELLY McGONIGAL, PhD, BESTSELLING AUTHOR OF
THE WILLPOWER INSTINCT

"Jessica is the 'friendo' who you always wished for . . . informed, encouraging, and always keeping it real. It's more than a good book. It's a great tool to take control of your health."

—SHANNON COHN, AWARD-WINNING DIRECTOR AND
PRODUCER OF *ENDO WHAT?* AND *BELOW THE BELT*

"If you're ready to define and live your best life rather than have endometriosis define you, you're in the right place."

—AVIVA ROMM, MD, AUTHOR OF *HORMONE INTELLIGENCE*

"Jessica Murnane's book is a must-read for people who suffer through endometriosis and for the people who love them."

—JUNE DIANE RAPHAEL, ACTRESS, SCREENWRITER,
AND COFOUNDER OF THE JANE CLUB

"Jessica so beautifully merged the science and research on pain and endometriosis with the real-world experiences of people living with endo. As a pelvic health PT, this will be one of my go-to resources for my patients living with endometriosis."

—DR. UCHENNA OSSAI, PHYSIOTHERAPIST, SEX COUNSELOR,
AND FOUNDER OF YOUSEELOGIC

"Jessica approaches this subject as she does everything: with curiosity and compassion, extensive research and a belief in the integration of modern allopathic med healthy lifestyle habits."

—MOZHAN MARNÒ, ACTRESS AND WR

"Endometriosis can break a person down—physically, emotionally. But there's hope in this book! I'm so glad that I *finally* have a book to help my patients with endometriosis."

—WILL BULSIEWICZ, MD, MSCI, *NEW YORK TIMES*
BESTSELLING AUTHOR OF *FIBER FUELED*

KNOW YOUR ENDO

An Empowering Guide to Health and Hope with Endometriosis

—

JESSICA MURNANE

AVERY

an imprint of Penguin Random House LLC

New York

AVERY

an imprint of Penguin Random House LLC
penguinrandomhouse.com

Most Avery books are available at special quantity discounts for bulk purchase for sales promotions, premiums, fund-raising, and educational needs. Special books or book excerpts also can be created to fit specific needs. For details, write Special Markets@penguinrandomhouse.com.

Library of Congress Cataloging-in-Publication Data

Names: Murnane, Jessica, author.
Title: Know your endo: an empowering guide to health and hope with endometriosis / Jessica Murnane.
Description: New York: Avery, an imprint of Penguin Random House LLC, [2021] | Includes index.
Identifiers: LCCN 2020040739 (print) | LCCN 2020040740 (ebook) | ISBN 9780593189832 (paperback) | ISBN 9780593189849 (ebook)
Subjects: LCSH: Endometriosis—Popular works. | Endometriosis—Treatment—Popular works. | Women—Health and hygiene—Popular works.
Classification: LCC RG483.E53 M87 2021 (print) | LCC RG483.E53 (ebook) | DDC 618.1/42—dc23
LC record available at https://lccn.loc.gov/2020040739
LC ebook record available at https://lccn.loc.gov/2020040740
p. cm.

Printed in the United States of America
1st Printing

Book design by Silverglass

FOR BONUS

CONTENTS

INTRODUCTION

At the beginning of this year, I had a "Celebrate Your Wins" party at my house. If you've never heard of a Celebrate Your Wins party before, that makes sense, because I made it up. So, let me explain a little. I invited my nearest and dearest (and some people I wanted to get to know better) over to my house for a big potluck to celebrate *us*. A lot of my friends had some rough times the previous year, and I thought we could use a party to focus on all the good stuff, too. So, when each guest came through the door, I handed them some sticky notes and a big fat marker and told them they had to write something they accomplished that they were proud of (a.k.a. their "win").

I'm not sure if you've ever tried this exercise before—to actually sit down and say why you're awesome and celebrate an accomplishment, without being allowed to follow it up with an apology for bragging or a "but it's not really that big of a deal!"—but it's not always an easy thing to do. Some of my friends' eyes got really wide when I handed them their sticky notes, like I had asked them to do something unimaginable. Others said they needed a drink first to get some courage to do it. And a few confidently grabbed the pad, sat down, and then gave me a "Help!" look from across the room. Eventually everyone wrote something down, and I took all the "wins" and stuck them on the wall together. Throughout the night, I'd stop the music and yell out a handful of wins from the wall, and we all cheered as loud as we could for that person's win.

In case you're nosey (like me) and wondering what some of the sticky notes said, here's a sampling: *"I stood up for myself,"* *"I decided to go to culinary school,"* *"I showed up for my dad,"* *"Had my best year in my business!,"* *"Woke up every day and tried again,"* and *"I've flossed my teeth every day for three months."* As the party was winding down, my friend and I stood in front of the wall with all the wins, smiling and taking them all in. She asked me, "Which one is yours?" I pointed to the one that read, *"I'm writing my dream book."* She looked at me a little surprised and told me that she knew I was writing another book but that I'd never mentioned anything about it being my "dream." I grinned really big and told her it was a huge dream come true for me and ended it there. That night, I didn't really feel like sharing more. Maybe because I wasn't sure if she'd totally get it, or maybe because I knew I'd get emotional and didn't think a crying host at such a positive party was a good look.

But I do want to share why it's my dream with *you.* Maybe because I know that you'll get it, and maybe because the emotions are already flowing (I've cried more happy and sad tears than I can count while writing and researching this book). But yes, writing this book is my dream. And I'm not going to apologize for bragging or downplay it by saying that it's not a big deal. Because it is a big deal.

A decade ago, my life didn't feel worth living anymore because of my endometriosis. It's such a complicated feeling to explain, because it wasn't that I wanted to die, but I really didn't want to live the current life I had, either. During the most painful weeks, I would obsessively fantasize about being in a sleep coma. In this coma, my body and mind would shut down and I'd fall into the deepest and most peaceful sleep of all time. My body would finally wake up when it didn't hurt anymore. I remember thinking that this deep sleep would mean I'd miss birthdays, weddings, big life events, and maybe even years of my life. But it would all be worth it to not feel my pain and sadness anymore and to no longer be a burden to the people who cared for me. I rationally knew this hibernation-like state wasn't a real possibility, but looking back, I think fantasizing about it gave my brain an alternate solution to the dark one lingering below the surface—the thought of not wanting to be alive at all. It was so hard to fathom that I would be in pain every single month, year after year—that I just wasn't sure this was a life worth living.

I also felt like I was living a double life. There was the me whom everyone saw—the person with an amazing husband, the kind of family and friends who would drop everything to help me, and an incredibly fun and ever-evolving career. I was driven, I wrote down my goals every year, and I was always up for new adventures. But then there was the other side of me that no one saw—the person who cried on the bathroom floor, who wondered if there was even a point to writing down those goals, and the person who didn't want to be awake anymore. I was sad and felt so desperately alone that it was hard to know what to do. But even those feelings were confusing. Because how did I have the right to be sad when I had such a great life? How dare I feel alone when I had so many people who loved me? This shame and guilt only made me feel worse. It got to a point where I had lost all hope that I'd ever live a "normal" life again.

My pain and symptoms became so severe that my doctor gave me two options: a hysterectomy or drug-hormone therapy. It was an easy decision for me: I picked the hysterectomy. Drugs felt temporary, and I just wanted all the parts that were causing me so much pain out of my body. I also didn't know back then that a hysterectomy didn't guarantee being pain-free. I was in such a dark place that I didn't want to wake up each day, and somehow a hysterectomy sounded easier than what I was going through. I felt so confident and relieved with the decision.

But then, like some sort of Hallmark-movie miracle, an angel-friend intervened. She emailed me a message that was the single most important one I think I'll ever receive. That email didn't even include a note, just a single link, the same way a friend quickly sends a link to a cute kitten video or a celebrity gossip story. But that single link changed my whole world. It led me to the first tool that finally helped me manage my endometriosis and changed my entire life. It sounds so easy breezy now . . . *my friend sent me a link and I wanted to be alive again!* But it wasn't that simple. I actually had zero faith it would work. If this tool was so life-changing, why didn't my doctors tell me about it? But my friend was nice enough to send it, so I agreed to try it for a few weeks. I was going to get a hysterectomy anyway, so what did I have to lose?

Within weeks of using this tool, my pain started to fade. Within months, the fog of my depression started to lift and many of my symptoms disappeared. After trying everything under the sun to feel better (surgery, legal drugs, not-so-legal drugs, and therapy), I had finally found something that worked to manage my pain and symptoms. That tool led to another and that led to another until my mind was completely cracked open with a new way of living. I actually felt like a brand-new me.

Actually, not a completely new me. Because even in my darkest and most painful times, my empathy, creativity, curiosity, drive, and love for my family and friends were still there. But my pain and depression buried them all so deep inside that I didn't feel like I could fully access those parts of me anymore. And now, I could.

Did all my cramps vanish forever? No. Do I still have endo? Yes. But, for the first time ever, I actually felt like I was in control of my endo and not the other way around. I became more confident, felt safer in my body, and my friends even said I became nicer. (Hey! Studies show that chronic pain can change your personality, which is something we'll be discussing in the chapters ahead.) I felt better than I ever had before. To my doctor's shock, I told her I wouldn't be getting the hysterectomy after all.

It's been ten years, and I still can't believe where I am today. I managed to climb out of the darkest time of my life and lived to tell about it. I was able to learn to manage my endo and truly find myself again. My endo no longer defines who I am. Standing where I am today (as in

I can literally stand up during my period—a big win), it truly feels like a dream come true.

But that's *not* why this is my dream book.

This book is my dream because my greatest hope is that by teaching you the same tools that changed my life, you might be able to live more of your dreams, too.

Maybe your dream right now is getting out of bed. It might be going back to work again. It might be moving your body more. It might be feeling less alone. It might be finding the confidence to speak up and advocate for yourself. It might be traveling more or just being able to hang with family and friends. During our time together, you might even discover a dream you didn't know you had or dig out the ones that got buried deep inside because of your pain. Will there be roadblocks and limitations to some of them? Maybe. But that doesn't mean we need to give up on *all* of them. That's the cool thing about dreams: we can change them, approach them in new ways, and have them meet us where we are.

Whatever your dreams are, all I want in this world is for you to get to a place where endo is no longer in the way of them—a place where we can celebrate *your* wins. So, one day, when we have our giant Celebrate Your Endo Wins Party, you'll be ready to write yours down, slap them up on the wall, and listen to us cheer for you.

I'm ready if you are.

With love, Jessica

A Few Things I Want You to Know before You Begin

1. The tools you're about to learn in the pages of this book are management practices, not treatments for endometriosis. These tools are not a cure and they will not stop your endo from growing. I wish it were as simple as "a green smoothie a day keeps the endo away!" but unfortunately, that's not how it works.

    While these tools are not a cure, they do have the potential to have a powerful impact on your life. After finishing this book, you might feel like you finally understand how to manage your endometriosis. You might feel better than you have in a very long time. But no matter how good you feel, you must continue to get checkups with your doctor. This means getting your annual exams, checking in when things don't feel right, and, for some, continuing (or asking for the first time) to get ultrasounds. I believe so strongly in the power of these tools, but I also believe strongly in the power of modern medicine. You don't need to choose one or the other. In fact, I believe they work best in tandem.

2. As you make your way through this book, please remember that we're all at different stages when it comes to managing our endometriosis, and we all have different levels of pain and

symptoms. A lot of this information might be things you already know and a breeze to incorporate into your life. But it also might be the first time you've ever heard any of these things, and you could find them challenging.

If you are someone who is pretty well-versed in these tools already, use this book as reinforcement and a high five to keep going. You can also use it as an opportunity to help others who are struggling. I see health and wellness book reviews all the time that say, "Nothing I didn't already know!" or "Heard it all before," which can be extremely discouraging to someone who is just starting out or overwhelmed on where to begin in the first place. If you already know a lot of this information, that's awesome. Now you have a chance to pay it forward and share this information and/or book with someone who has yet to discover it.

If you are someone who doesn't know a thing about endo or you have no clue how to begin to manage it, that's okay! It's never too late to get started, and that's why I wrote this book. I've spoken to so many people with endo who feel stupid or embarrassed for being in the dark for so long about their condition. *Why didn't they ask more questions? Why didn't they advocate for themselves better?* I received a message once from a woman who struggled for decades with her endo, and it wasn't until she visited my website that she discovered that fatigue was a symptom of endometriosis. This was a huge "aha" moment for her. She finally felt validated for all the years she struggled with her fatigue, and everything made more sense to her.

The changes I'm asking you to make in this book might not come easily at first. You might question if they are worth it and if there's any point in trying. They are worth it. Let's agree to ditch any feelings of shame or embarrassment for what you don't or didn't know. Let's also agree not to give yourself a hard time if they don't come easily for you in the beginning.

We all have to start somewhere. And you are starting here, right now.

3. Historically, endometriosis was seen as a "woman's condition," but not every person with endometriosis identifies as a woman. Throughout the book you will see that I use "person" instead of "woman" and "friendo" (friend with endo) instead of "endo sister" whenever I can. There are still some instances where I needed to use "woman/women" or female pronouns. You will also see these pronouns in some of the research and quotes from people I interviewed, but these are rare. Regardless of these instances, please know that inclusivity is important and everyone with endo matters to our community.

4. Throughout the book, you'll see friendos answering questions from the Endo Questionnaire I created (a riff on the famous Proust Questionnaire). You can find more of their answers and download your own questionnaire to share at knowyourendo.com /endoquestions.

Making Yourself a Priority

Before we dive into the ins and outs of endo and your tools, I want to make sure we're on the same page in terms of the mindset you'll need to approach this book. What I'm about to say might be something you've never allowed yourself to think before and might be hard to take in, but I need you to try your best to accept it. And that is: *if you're a person living with endometriosis, caring for yourself needs to be your number-one priority.*

I know what you might be thinking. *What about my job? My family? My school? My other responsibilities? Also, it sounds pretty selfish to put* my *care above everything else.* I understand that your plate might already be full of commitments and responsibilities. And when you have endo, just making it out of bed in the morning can feel like a part-time job. I also understand that so many of us have been dismissed or been made to feel small because of this condition. If you've been told time after time that your pain is in your head, that you're exaggerating, or that it can't really be *that* bad, why would you dare make the time and space to care for yourself?

But here's what I have to say to that . . .

If you're a person living with endometriosis, caring for yourself needs to be your number-one priority.

I want to be clear about what taking care of yourself means, because there's been a lot of "self-care" talk out there these days and that phrase has morphed over the years. "Self-care" has gone from a single act of kindness you can do for yourself to an entire industry full of products, services, and wellness experiences. It's exciting to see so many brands jump on board the self-care train, but the problem is that many of these products and services don't fit into the majority of our budgets or schedules. And for some, the new world of self-care practices can feel intimidating, overwhelming, confusing, or too weird to try in the first place.

So, we end up doing nothing for ourselves, don't think "self-care" is for us (or we're not worthy of it), and end up exactly where we are, feeling lousy.

First off, everyone is worthy of caring for themselves. The fact that you are reading this book tells me you know this (at least a little bit). And let's also be clear that I'm not suggesting that you neglect your family or job because you're too busy taking long baths, doing intensive skin treatments, and bingeing on all the latest wellness trends. I am suggesting that you spend the time you need to take care of you without feeling guilty about it. It's not selfish to take care of yourself when you're in pain. It's not selfish to want to be able to get out of bed. It's not selfish to want to be excited to wake up in the morning. And it's not selfish to want to feel good.

Second, caring for ourselves doesn't have to be so complicated and expensive. I'm not going to lie, I've definitely tried a lot of the fancy powders and potions, been on a retreat or two, and I enjoy some pricey workout classes from time to time. All of these things feel good at the time, but they're not practical or financially sustainable ways for me to practice caring for myself every single day. Instead I do my best to shut out all the unnecessary wellness and self-care marketing noise and focus on the fundamental tools for a healthy body and mind with endometriosis—these are the tools I'll be teaching you in this book.

In our time together, I will show you ways to care for yourself that are simple and practical and don't require you to invest half of your paycheck in the latest wellness trend. Most of the tools I'll be teaching you in this book are ones that require only two things: your body and an open mind.

I hope you're willing to make caring for yourself a priority, but if you're still not on board because you're worried about taking time away from your other responsibilities, please remember that when we are truly able to care for ourselves, we are able to inch closer to thriving in the other parts of our lives, and better care for those we love. Think about how much your pain and symptoms get in the way of your relationships, your work, and/or giving back to your community. Now think about how much more time you would have to give to them if you felt better.

What do you admire most about yourself living with endo?

Getting help. It took me twenty-eight years, but damn it . . . I finally got the message that my body was trying to tell me!

—Jamie Michelle Fox

Your New Endo Tool Kit

The tools you're about to discover were born from a course I designed called the Endo Tool Kit. When I set out to teach the course, I thought maybe it would be something I did a couple of times a year while I wrote another cookbook and taught cooking classes. But then I started to hear the transformations and success stories from people who took the course, and it was all I could think about! I wondered how I could dive even deeper into these tools and find more ways to support the endo community by teaching them. I realized I didn't want to write another cookbook; I wanted to write *this* book. And here we are.

Before we get to your new tools (and I swear we'll get to them in a minute!), I think it's important to remember that we all have very unique bodies, and endo can be a very complex condition. I wish I could promise that these tools will make all your pain and symptoms disappear completely and that you'll never need surgery (for the first time or ever again), but I can't. But what I can promise is that I am giving you all the information you need to feel empowered to be a better advocate for yourself and to never stop asking questions. To help you understand that the choices you make for your health and the way you talk to yourself *can* make a difference. To give you hope that it's possible to have more good days than bad. And most important, to know that you are not alone.

Here's How This Is Going to Work

At the beginning of this book, I'll be covering the ins and outs of endo, essentially a crash course in all things endometriosis—what it is, types of surgeries and treatments, sister diseases, and how it can impact your relationships, work, and mental/physical health. There will also be some places where you'll be asked to share more about you and your endo, too. It's important to read everything and not skip ahead. It's also important to grab a pen and write down your thoughts, whenever I ask you to. So much of what you'll be reading and writing will help you be better prepared for your new management plan ahead. It might also help you discover things you didn't know about yourself.

After you've finished your crash course in endo, you'll start learning and practicing one new management tool per week, for five weeks. Only one tool a week?! I know this might be difficult for all the type A personalities and overachievers out there (which is a lot of people with endo!). You might have gotten so good at doing it all and pushing through—despite your condition—that you want to do it all at once. But be patient and stick to one tool a week. This progressive plan gives you some room to breathe and dials back the pressure to be perfect at everything, all at once.

If you are not able to do the weeks consecutively, that's okay. Jump back in when you can! And if you feel like you need more time on a certain tool before you move on, stick with it. This is your endo to manage, and you know best what your mind and body can handle.

Your new tools:
Week One: Know Your Endo
Week Two: Stress Management
Week Three: Good Food
Week Four: Movement
Week Five: Kinder Home + Body

After learning these tools, we'll also dive into alternative medicine and therapies. I chose not to include these practices as part of your foundational tools because, depending on where you live or the budget you're working with, they might not all be available to you. Like I said, it's my mission to provide you with the most practical and accessible tools I can—ones that you can practice without even leaving your home.

————

After completing this book, you'll find that some of these tools will become nonnegotiables and will be used every day of your life. Others might take a back seat on certain days. For instance, for me, my Good Food tool is a nonnegotiable. It manages my pain the best. But there are times when I'm traveling or it's the first day of my period that my stress-management tools (moving my body or my calming hobbies) are not in the cards. And that's okay. I still have these tools in my belt, and I can pull them out whenever I need them.

One of the most exciting things about finding tools that work is the hope they bring. Most of us have experienced pretty hopeless days dealing with endo. And with that hopelessness, feelings of fear, anger, and sadness can be triggered inside us. Which only makes us feel worse. But what if you knew you had a tool in your back pocket that could make you feel even a little bit better? What if, on those painful days in bed, you knew that tomorrow was a new day because you had a tool that could help manage that fear, anger, and sadness better? The tools you'll be learning can slowly begin a change, not just to how you manage your endo, but how you approach each day.

Creating your new tool kit might not feel super easy in the beginning. You may have some guilt around it. You might be feeling so sad and in pain right now that it doesn't feel possible to see the light. Some of these concepts might be outside your comfort zone. You may have been conditioned to believe that everyone and everything (besides you) comes first. But you are a person with endo. Which automatically makes you stronger and more resilient. Remember, it is not selfish to want to take care of yourself—and that new habits take time.

———

Now that you're on board with making yourself a priority (or getting closer to believing this), there's one more thing you need to do before we get started. So please grab a pen, because you're going to be completing your first exercise in this next section. Here we go . . .

Defining Your Best

There was a time, after introducing all my diet and lifestyle tools, that I became obsessed with feeling "well." I wanted to be *perfect* at wellness, and I tried everything I could to achieve wellness perfection (which is impossible to do, by the way). I blew through hundreds of books, articles, and documentaries on the topic of inflammation, the perfect diet for my body, and period health. I got stool tests to make sure my gut—and all the critters in there—were healthy and happy. I did cleanses and colonics. I tried twenty different workouts and more than twenty different supplements, powders, and "magic" potions to see which my body liked best. It was a lot of trial and error, a lot of money, and, looking back, a lot of stress and pressure I put on myself to be this glowing poster child of perfect health. Not just endo health, *all* health.

I don't think there's anything wrong with wanting to try everything you can (within reason) to feel better. In fact, today I still use some of the products and practices I discovered during my perfectionism days. And I wouldn't be sitting here upright in this chair, writing this page, if I'd never tried the tools I'm sharing in this book. The problem was that when I was going overboard with all those cleanses and obsessing over all the information I could find, I was already feeling pretty great. Not just great—better than I had in the previous twenty years of my life. I was not only getting out of bed during my period, I was thriving. I felt more connected to my body. I was able to spend more time with family and friends, go on trips, and move my body (on my period!). But that wasn't enough.

After making initial changes to my diet and lifestyle and getting a little taste of feeling great, a.k.a. "my best," I wanted to push my best even further. I was on a mission to get rid of every ounce of inflammation in my body, never have cramps again, and figure out how to live a fatigue-free life. I had been so successful with the changes I'd already made, I wanted more. *What if my best could be even better?*

I don't think I'm alone in this pursuit. We're constantly hit with the phrase "your best" when it comes to our health. You'll find it on the covers of books and magazines, in ads, and on social media. I'm not opposed to this phrase, but if we're going to be talking about feeling "your best," we need to narrow in on the "your" part of this phrase. Not *yours* compared to someone else's. Especially not *yours* compared to someone who does not have endo. Just and only *yours*. There seems to be this unspoken universal standard of what "your best" means, and this standard is constantly changing with new diets, workout trends, wellness products, and fashion cycles that dictate what *your* most desired body should be.

Which makes it incredibly confusing to know what to do. It can paralyze us from making any change at all because we're afraid of it not working, or we don't even know where to start. Melissa, a friendo from Canada, told me she really struggles with this big time. She told me, "There's so much that we can do. There are so many different aspects that sometimes I just feel super overwhelmed, and I don't know where to start. What's the hierarchy? What's the foundation of where you start? How do you build an action plan of what to try? I know doing an elimination diet or keeping a journal of stuff would help. But I don't do any of that stuff, because I'm just so overwhelmed with all the things that I should be doing right." I've heard so many people in the endo community echo the same feelings as Melissa. And it's why I wanted to write this book: to give people a new foundation, a place to start.

While Melissa didn't know where to start, there's also the set of people (like me) who try everything under the sun and go down a path of unrealistic expectations and wellness perfectionism, which can turn into a very unhappy and confusing place to live. After trying everything I did, I was definitely confused. I was also really tired. And I'm not talking about the fatigue from my endometriosis. I had a whole new kind of fatigue: wellness fatigue. Every single week, I was obsessively trying to refine and readjust my diet, supplements, workouts, and products to get even more out of my body. After a couple of years of this, I hit a wall. I remember I had a good cry session when it happened. I cried about how sick I was of trying so hard. I was actually annoyed at hearing my own voice talk about "wellness." I felt suffocated by how much all of it occupied my thoughts. I knew I needed to make a change

In order to change, I needed to accept what "my best" was while living with endo. But I didn't want to do that. Because I knew that my best was probably someone else's worst. I also might never be able to make my best any better. My best would mean never running a marathon on my period. It was having the energy to get out of bed and walk

What is your endo motto?

Consistency heals.

—Daphne Javitch

around the block. It would mean never wearing only a panty liner on the first few days of my period. It was wearing an overnight pad *and* leak-proof underwear. And it would mean never having spontaneous and wild sex in whatever position I wanted. It was being strategic and careful in bed, so it didn't hurt too much.

Melissa told me she struggled with this, too. She constantly wonders how much of her pain and symptoms she just might have to accept as part of her life living with endo.

I get it. Acceptance feels like defeat. Growing up, I was taught that if you work hard and stay positive, you can accomplish anything you set your mind to. My family didn't invent this idea, of course. There are hundreds of books, podcasts, and memes devoted to the idea that *Anything is possible! Smile and the world smiles with you! Work hard and everything else will fall into place! All you need is dedication to make it happen!* Working hard and staying positive were at the core of my belief system about living a good life. I applied these mantras to my school, career, and really everything I did, including my health.

But not too long ago, I began to question this idea. What if anything and everything wasn't possible with endo? What if I had done all I could? What if I could stop trying to make my best better? I felt like a huge Negative Nelly even considering this. All of those same books, podcasts, and memes told me to *Never give up, no matter what! Your destiny is in your hands! You can manifest anything!* But when I really thought about the life I wanted, I knew that my quest for perfect health wasn't bringing me up—it was bringing me down. I also realized that I really had come a long way, and I needed to celebrate that more. It felt liberating to focus on the tools that I knew worked and stop trying to be so perfect.

Time to Begin

We are never going to live in a perfect body, because it's not possible. But what we can do is define what success and "your best" means for your body. If we never measure or define this success, how will we know when we're actively achieving it? And this definition might change over time. At the end of this book, you might completely shift what "your best" means to you, and right now you might have no idea what that looks like. And that's okay. We're just getting started. When I got real with my best, I was able to admit that the obsession with never having an ounce of inflammation in my body again was unrealistic, *but* lowering my inflammation to the point where my joints didn't hurt was totally doable. Never having a single period cramp again? Probably not going to happen. *But* I was able to manage my cramps enough that I could work, cook, and move my body during my period. Which was huge. And a fatigue-free life? Also, nada. I'm just going to be a little more tired on some days because of my endo. It's nothing I did wrong, *but* on those tired days, I allow myself to sleep an extra twenty minutes, without judgment.

And as we kick off this book, I want you to start celebrating your wins more and also track how far you've come already. Some of my endo wins include being able to pick up my son from school on the first day of my period and no longer crying on the bathroom floor. Sometimes when we're in the thick of it, we forget how much progress we've already made. You might have a lot of endo wins already, or you're someone who is hurting so bad right now that it makes you cry thinking about me making you come up with one. So, if you don't feel like you have any right now, that's okay. The following page will be here for you when you're ready. You're also allowed to write down wins you want to accomplish, too.

I will never be perfect at wellness, and neither will you. But it feels so good to accept my endo best and celebrate the wins that I've worked so hard to accomplish. Acceptance is not defeat. It's also not a pass to never try or an excuse to lie in bed and call it quits. It's permission to define success for your own very unique body. To be kinder to yourself. To say goodbye to perfectionism. And shamelessly brag about how far you've come or what you're about to do.

Now You.

Have you struggled with doing too much or being too overwhelmed to start managing your endo?

_____

_____

_____

_____

_____

_____

Share what "your best" looks and feels like living with endo.

_____

_____

_____

_____

_____

_____

What are some of your endo wins?

_____

_____

_____

_____

_____

_____

_____

If you can't think of any, what are some you are hoping for?

_____

_____

_____

_____

_____

_____

The Ins and Outs of Endo

Growing up, I remember my mom unbuttoning her jeans whenever she got home and walked through the door. She would leave them unbuttoned as she caught up with friends on the phone and cooked us dinner, and really until she put us to bed each night. I never asked her why she did this. I just thought that was what happened to moms at the end of the day because their stomachs were so bloated. From time to time, I'd see little blood stains on the back of her pants and figured it was normal to have your period leak through your pants. I also saw her struggle to keep up at times, and she was really tired a lot—which didn't seem totally crazy because she had four kids to care for, almost entirely on her own (my stepdad was in the military and was deployed for up to six months at a time). She had bladder issues, which again, didn't seem totally out of the norm when you've given birth to four kids. She never complained to us about her period pain or the other health issues she experienced. But as time went on, her period pain and symptoms got increasingly worse, and she opted to have a hysterectomy at the age of forty-six.

When I started having periods of my own, we didn't talk much about the pain or the symptoms I had. Witnessing what my mom experienced each month, I just assumed period pain was our family's norm, so there really wasn't much to discuss. My mom never once questioned or complained about picking me up from school because of my period pain or when my own blood leaked through my pants. And she always had Aleve and a heating pad on standby when I needed it. Again, this was our norm.

It wasn't until my sister and I were diagnosed that my mom first heard the word "endometriosis." Looking back, I have a hard time understanding why no doctor had ever mentioned endometriosis to her before (not even the doctor who performed her hysterectomy), when she was clearly struggling with all the classic symptoms.

But she's not alone.

I spoke with Lynette, a yoga instructor, who was diagnosed at fifty-three years old. Before being diagnosed, Lynette says she hadn't really heard about endo, either. She told me that when she was in her twenties, she had a neighbor with endo and remembers her neighbor's doctor urging her to hurry up and have kids. But other than that, she said she didn't know anything about it. Fast-forward thirty years, when at her annual exam, her doctors found a mass in her colon. After they biopsied the mass, they told her, "Well, it's an endometrial mass." And she told them, "But I don't have endometriosis." Lynette not only had endometriosis, but she later learned her endo had caused irreparable damage to her body.

Lynette's doctors thought they could laparoscopically remove the colon mass, but as they began the surgery, her doctors discovered that many of Lynette's organs had fused together because of her endometriosis (her surgeon described her endo as "Gorilla Glue"). What was supposed to be a laparoscopic procedure turned into a six-hour surgery where Lynette says they opened her up from "above my navel to below my C-section incisions" to remove the endometriosis and perform a double bowel resection. She's also had a hysterectomy and two subsequent bowel surgeries, and she fears there could be more in the future.

———

Why had her severe case of endometriosis gone undetected for so long? For starters, Lynette said she was able to have two children in her mid-twenties—"anybody I had heard of who had endo had trouble having kids, and I had zero problem having kids." And in her thirties, she said, "I remember telling my doctors at every single annual exam that I was having horrible periods, horrible cramping, and heavy bleeding." She also had terrible rectal pain, pelvic floor pain, and pain during intercourse during certain times of her cycle. And she said, "I was even diagnosed with fibromyalgia when I was in my early thirties." She told me that in her midforties things began to escalate—and again her doctors never brought up endometriosis and told her it was just perimenopause. "I went in every year for my annual exam like I was supposed to. I had my Pap smear, and every year they just put 'dysmenorrhea' on the chart, sent me out with the pills, and didn't address it at all. I was completely dismissed for more than two decades."

Over the course of my interview with Lynette, she sounded calm and more positive than I'd expected for someone who had gone through what she did. So, I asked her how she's feeling emotionally about her experience over the last few years. She said that she really struggles with anxiety and depression and is seeing a therapist who works with people who have chronic illnesses and medical traumas. And she shared, "As we speak, I'm supposed to go get blood work, and I'm putting it off because I can't do it. Going in and being handled by doctors, I've just sort of had enough. It brings everything back to the surface for me."

Lynette says she tries to stay positive, and after she was diagnosed she went on a one-woman campaign to tell all the women in her life to "make sure somebody pays attention to you." She told me that so much of the endo discussion is around women in their childbearing years and their fertility. But Lynette wants her story to be an example of what happens when a person's symptoms are ignored for decades. "The results were, for me, catastrophic. My life is permanently altered."

Getting Diagnosed

I wish Lynette's and my mom's stories were unique, but they're not. It's estimated that 176 million people worldwide have endometriosis. *And yet* the average time it takes from the onset of symptoms to receiving a diagnosis is between eight and ten years. Some people may go through years of infertility treatments and never receive a diagnosis. Laparoscopy is the only way to truly diagnose endometriosis (which we'll talk more about in a minute), but many may never have that diagnostic surgery. *And* 75 percent of people with endometriosis will be misdiagnosed—with everything from appendicitis and ovarian cancer to irritable bowel syndrome (IBS) and/or a sexually transmitted disease.

Whether it took you two years or two decades, chances are you remember the age you were (or the exact date) when you were diagnosed. Maybe that's the day that you finally felt heard. Or the day you finally had proof that the pain wasn't in your head. Or the day that you finally understood why you had so much fatigue, GI problems, fertility issues, back pain, and painful sex. Or all of the above. The day you were diagnosed *is* a very significant day. But that day can also come with a lot of emotional questions: *Why did it take me so long to be diagnosed? Why didn't my family and friends believe my pain? Why is this the first time I've even heard the word "endometriosis"? And what does my future look like living with an incurable condition?*

Years after being diagnosed you might still be asking yourself those questions. You might still not truly understand your condition. And that's not uncommon. Nearly all the people with endo whom I've interviewed and talked to over the years say they were relieved to get a diagnosis. But after that diagnosis, they still felt in the dark about it. And the majority blamed themselves for not asking their doctor more questions or pushing to get diagnosed sooner.

If you're someone who blames themselves or feels weak or stupid that reading this book is the first time you're learning more about endo, take a moment and do this exercise with me.

Start by thinking of a friend or family member you love, someone you truly care about in your life. Now imagine that person suffering for years with pain and discomfort but being told that their pain was in their head, they were being dramatic, or they simply needed to toughen up. No matter how hard they tried, they still struggled to go to work or school, had to cancel plans because of their pain, and felt hopeless and alone.

Now, imagine that person, after seeing a handful (maybe two handfuls) of doctors, finally finding their way to a doctor who was willing to investigate their pain and symptoms further. That doctor agreed to perform exploratory surgery. It went "well" and now the person you love is sitting on top of a table in an examination room or maybe lying in a hospital bed just out of surgery, waiting to hear the results.

Their doctor walks in (or a doctor they have never met before, because their doctor is off that day), telling them they do have something wrong with them, an incurable condition. The doctor tells the person you love that they did their best to remove the disease but can't promise it won't come back. In fact, it probably will. And there's not that much they can do about it.

They also say that birth control could help manage their pain and symptoms, but in the same breath they casually advise them to start thinking about getting pregnant sooner rather than later if they ever want kids. Alternatively, a hysterectomy might be in their future, but they could also try hormone treatments to force their body into menopause to see if that helps first. The doctor needs to get to the next patient, so the doctor quickly runs through these options, without sharing the side effects or other lifestyle-management tools they could try. And the doctor never really explains exactly what this newly diagnosed condition is or why they have it in the first place. The doctor tells the person you love to think about their options and come back to see the doctor again in a few months.

As the doctor walks out, they say *again* that they really should start thinking about getting pregnant if they want kids. The person you love sits or lies there alone—confused, in shock, and not sure how to process the information they just heard.

Does this story sound familiar? This scenario is the story I hear time and time again from people with endo on their diagnosis day. But what happened when you imagined that scenario happening to someone else, someone you love? You probably didn't blame that person for not asking more questions, or see them as weak for not pushing to be heard, or stupid for not trying to understand their condition until reading this book. You most likely had compassion for them. And I hope you are able to extend that same compassion to yourself. Because if this is your story, too, it's not your fault.

———

Casey Berna, an endometriosis counselor and social worker who actively fights for endometriosis care reform, says, "The current standards of care and the ignorance of the gynecological community surrounding endometriosis is causing medical trauma to patients. It's causing physical trauma, emotional trauma, delay in the diagnosis, dismissal of pain, misdiagnosis, and repeating treatments that are ineffective. And it's a huge problem that the majority of patients do not have access to quality care or access to quality information."

If this has not been your experience, and the first doctor you saw believed your pain, diagnosed you at a young age, took the time to explain endometriosis to you, and gave you other resources for management options (outside of hormones), please share your doctor's number with every person you know who has a period! Because this is rare.

And no, I'm not in the business of villainizing doctors. Because there are some pretty amazing ones out there fighting for funding and research for endometriosis and taking the time to educate their patients with compassion. Shannon Cohn, the endometriosis activist and founder of *Endo What?*, shares that "most doctors are good people trying to do a good job. Most." But she says the majority are "simply not being educated properly about this condition. It has not been made a priority historically. Women's health and below-the-belt issues have not been a priority in medical school or medical practices. The education has not been there as far as helping doctors identify the real symptomatic profile." She says after you're diagnosed, you enter a "whole other vortex" about finding the right treatments, and doctors are just not told how to help you do this.

It's okay to be mad at the way you were treated. It's okay to be sad. It's okay to feel whatever emotions you have about trying to find answers and convincing someone to believe you.

But here's the thing. None of us can go back in time and change our diagnosis day or how many years it took to get diagnosed. You can't change how you were mistreated in the past or that no one ever sat down to explain your condition to you. You can't change that your family and friends said it was "all in your head." And you can't change the fact that you have endometriosis.

What you can change is what happens next.

In the pages ahead, you'll truly get to know the ins and outs of endometriosis. And with this information, I'm hoping you'll be able to empower yourself to get the best care you're able to receive. Will this always be easy? No. Even with this information, you still might feel nervous or too overwhelmed to speak up. You might still have people question your pain and symptoms. It might take some practice to push for the care you deserve, and you might not do it perfectly every time. But you will be armed with everything you need to start. For a lot of people with endo, this is a huge first step. If you've made giant strides already and think you know everything about endo, please keep reading. You might discover something new or learn how you can better advocate for those who aren't yet ready or able to.

Dr. Karli Goldstein, an endometriosis excision surgeon specialist who had endo herself, was an invaluable resource for the information in this chapter and will help guide you through the medical questions. She's one of those great doctors fighting the good fight as an excision surgeon in the operating room and is working hard for better care and more compassion for every patient with endo.

Let's get started.

What Is Endometriosis?

Endometriosis in an inflammatory condition in which endometrial-like tissue (similar to the tissue that lines the uterus and is shed during menstruation) is found in other places in the body. It usually involves the ovaries, the bowel, or the tissue lining your pelvis, though sometimes it can spread beyond the pelvic region, including, but not limited to, the appendix, diaphragm, and lungs.

What Are the Symptoms?

Very painful periods (pelvic pain, cramping, lower-back and abdominal pain)*

Pain during ovulation or two weeks after your period

Leg pain or neuralgia (nerve sensations) associated with your cycle

Hip pain and/or back pain

Shoulder/chest pain or shortness of breath with your cycle

Pain during or after sex

---

* Not everyone with endometriosis has painful periods. Some people experience periods without pain but then experience other symptoms the rest of the month.

Thick blood clots (often dark) with your period

Painful bowel movements or painful urination

Excessive bleeding

Fatigue and chronic pain

Diarrhea and constipation

Bloating

Nausea and vomiting

Urinary frequency, retention, or urgency

Allergies and other immune-related issues

Infertility and pregnancy loss (though many people can still
have children)

Endometriosis symptoms can begin at a person's first period and can
also change over time. Some people may not experience symptoms until
many years after starting their first period. And some who take birth
control as contraception for years do not notice symptoms until they
stop using it. You might experience one or all of these symptoms, but the
number of symptoms you experience does not always correlate to the
stage of your condition or how disruptive endometriosis is to your life.

How Is Endo Diagnosed?

You must have a diagnostic laparoscopy with a biopsy of the tissue to
have a definitive endometriosis diagnosis. A laparoscopy is done using a
laparoscope (small lighted instrument) through an incision near the
belly button and smaller incisions for the surgical instruments.

I have heard from so many friendos over the years who say that they
received their diagnosis via imaging (ultrasound or MRI), an annual
exam, or blood test—but these are not a true diagnosis. Dr. Goldstein
says, "You can have a high index of suspicion from an ultrasound or an
exam, but the only real true diagnosis is actually on biopsy where a

What do you wish everyone knew about living with endometriosis?

I wish that everyone knew that endometriosis is not just a "(rich) white woman's disease." It affects people of all racial backgrounds.

—Samantha Denae

pathologist looks under the microscope for endometrial glands and stroma that are visualized in the tissue."

Friendos have also told me that their doctors diagnosed them after seeing a cyst via imaging but did not further investigate with a laparoscopy or advise the cyst be removed (even when it was a large one). Dr. Goldstein says you can see cysts via an ultrasound, and they could turn out to be endometrioma (chocolate cysts). This, again, is a good index of suspicion of endometriosis. But this is not a diagnosis.

She says that every now and then, even with the best ultrasound or MRI, the fluid in a cyst can turn out to not be endometriotic fluid. Again, imaging is not a foolproof diagnosis.

"If the cyst is a chocolate cyst and it's sizable," Dr. Goldstein says, "we don't recommend watching and waiting forever. Why? Because frequently those can leak, can cause adhesions, and cause more damage later. The bowel can become adherent to the ovary, and the ovary can attach to the uterus or tubes and create dense, thick adhesions and destruction. What could have been a straightforward cyst removal can turn into much deeper surgery if not managed on time."

Not to mention, a ruptured cyst can cause severe pain. I'm not sure what the medical terminology is for "hurts like hell," but from experience, I can tell you that a ruptured cyst can feel like the worst period you've ever experienced plus someone putting a blowtorch on your insides and then stabbing those insides with a sharp knife. I've heard of doctors telling endo patients with 6cm (2.36-inch) and 8cm (3.15-inch) cysts that it's perfectly fine to leave that cyst alone—if it ruptures, it won't cause them too much pain. This is not true. Ask anyone who has had a ruptured cyst, and they will tell you otherwise.

What Do the Stages of Endometriosis Mean?

The stage of your disease does not always reflect the level of pain or how many symptoms you experience. At the time of this writing, the Endometriosis Foundation of America is proposing to change these stages to be more descriptive, because each stage has so many variations and does not account for where lesions are located or the patient's pain. For instance, you could have Stage II and have more pain than someone with Stage IV, simply based on where the lesions are located in your body.

Here are the current classifications of stages:

Stage I: Minimal with few superficial implants

Stage II: Mild with more and deeper implants

Stage III: Moderate with many deep implants, small cysts on one or both ovaries, presence of filmy adhesions

Stage IV: Severe with many deep implants, large cysts on one or both ovaries, many dense adhesions

Is It Genetic?

Dr. Goldstein says that we still don't have a definitive answer to this question, but there is more evidence to prove that there are genetic factors related to endometriosis. People who have a relative with endo are five to seven times more likely to have it.

Keep in mind that so many of our mothers, grandmothers, aunts, and older generations were likely never diagnosed. Endo was talked about even *less* during their reproductive years, and a lot of them suffered without knowing why. This is another good reason to speak up— to share your pain, symptoms, and everything you know about endo, with all the women in your life. No matter their age. They may have been suffering in silence for years, and sharing could help them not only find answers but also feel less alone.

What Causes Endometriosis to Happen?

Dr. Goldstein says that it's complicated and most likely multifactorial, but there is funding and research going into the discovery of why it happens. She explains that if there was a one-shot way this developed, then it would be easier to develop a therapy or drug to target and stop it. She went on to say, "There are multiple theories that include genetic origins or mutations, Mullerian/embryonic development abnormalities, retrograde menstruation or stem cell metaplasia, environmental toxins, and immune dysfunction."

As Dr. Goldstein says, it's complicated, and she believes it is most likely a combination of multiple theories. But research and funding *are* happening, and it's hopeful we'll have answers in the years to come.

Is Adenomyosis the Same as Endometriosis?

Adenomyosis is not endometriosis, but they are often called sister diseases or of a similar family. Adenomyosis is when endometrial tissue grows within the muscle walls of the uterus instead of only within the endometrial cavity. Adenomyosis can cause extremely painful cramping and dysfunctional bleeding with dark thick clots during a period, which is very similar to endo.

People who have adenomyosis are more likely to have endometriosis, but if you have endo, it doesn't mean you have adenomyosis. But if you have adenomyosis, you most likely have endometriosis elsewhere in the body. Dr. Goldstein notes, "Adenomyosis, or a solitary location of it referred to as adenomyoma, is often confused with fibroids when imaging is done." So, it's important to find an endo specialist with knowledge of adenomyosis who will be able to help you create a treatment and management plan that is best for you.

Getting Treatment

What Is the Best Treatment for Endo?

Excision surgery is recommended over any other surgical methods, such as laser ablation surgery. Excision surgery gets to the root of the inflammatory tissue, whereas ablation surgery burns and attempts to treat the most superficial layer of the disease. Because ablation is not truly excising the disease, Dr. Goldstein shares that this is why many patients say their surgery "didn't work." In many cases their surgeon "couldn't burn along the ureter, they couldn't burn around the ovary, they couldn't burn around the bowel or the bladder. And sometimes they're just leaving 60 to 70 percent of the lesions untreated." They are only getting the ones that are safe to burn.

Dr. Goldstein calls this an "incomplete surgery," and unfortunately it can result in continuing pain and associated issues. She says many patients who have ablation surgery can have increased pain after surgery. This can happen when lesions are overlying small nerves coursing under the peritoneal layer—when you burn the outer layer, it can create fibrotic scar tissue and even hurt the nerve below. With excision surgery, the surgeon not only removes diseased and damaged tissue but can also reconstruct organs and restore their functionality. This is not to say that all your pain and symptoms will vanish forever after one excision surgery, but it does give you a greater chance of finding relief and increasing the amount and/or length of time between surgeries in the future.

Excision surgery is deemed the "gold standard" of treatment and diagnosis for endo, but unfortunately it is not an option for many. Not only are some patients not told that there is an alternative to ablation surgery, but even if they have this knowledge, it's not an affordable option for everyone—with or without insurance.

Shannon Cohn explains that everything you would go to see a doctor for has a CPT code. In the United States, this is the code the doctor uses when billing insurance to show what surgical or diagnostic service they performed. As of this writing, an endometriosis surgery has only one CPT code, whether a doctor spent thirty minutes doing an ablation surgery burning away a few lesions or six hours excising thirty lesions, repairing or reconstructing organs, and/or bringing in other specialists to assist in the surgery.

Dr. Goldstein shares that excision surgery can be a highly complex surgery that has much higher risk involved than a typical laparoscopic gynecological surgery. And a surgeon's malpractice insurance is higher in order to cover this liability they take on. She shares that these surgeries are a team effort, and this disease can humble even the best of surgeons. Yet, both ablation and excision surgeries are reimbursed the same. This is problematic. Depending on the complexity of the surgery, a doctor who is performing a skilled excision surgery might only be able to perform one to three surgeries a day. The compensation from the insurance company for this one surgery is not enough to keep the lights on in their practice. This is why skilled excision surgeons are generally out of network.

While some excision specialists do their best to perform a handful of pro bono cases a year or help navigate payment plans and reimbursements from insurance companies with their patients, it's a much larger systemic issue that is going to take time to change. Heather Guidone, a board-certified patient advocate who has been working for more than two decades to change these systems, says that she is hopeful. "For a really long time, decades even, it has been shouting into the void," she said. "But we're seeing more surgeons and endo specialists really getting involved, pushing back against the system, and advocating for their patients. There are robust efforts going into the coding. There are robust efforts going into the guidelines. And when one changes, it changes the other. I do know that enough noise is being made by enough people that the AMA [American Medical Association] and the ACOG [American College of Obstetricians and Gynecology] are starting to take notice."

What if I Had an Ablation Surgery and Feel Great?
Did I Do Something Wrong?

No, and it's incredible if you feel good! Heather says, "This condition is not one size fits all. You may get an ablation with a local ob-gyn, and she may burn a few surface lesions off. You may feel really good. Some folks do really well with that. That's the reality. Some folks will have minor areas of the disease. So, it is difficult to say, 'Yes, everyone has to have excision.' Of course, we would love that. But the reality is, there is a lot of privilege that goes into that kind of care. And recognizing that, we have to do the best we can with what we have to work with."

How Do I Find a Good Endo Doctor or Surgeon?

This is easier said than done because not everyone has insurance, not everyone has the means to find a specialist, not everyone lives in a city where there is more than one option for care, and not everyone feels confident enough to see a doctor in the first place.

A good place to start is by checking in with your fellow endo community to see which doctors they had a good experience with, whether that's joining an online endo community group or reaching out to friendos to ask for resources that have helped them. If budget is an issue, you can try contacting an endometriosis foundation to see if they are able to financially assist you or if they know of doctors who will work on a sliding scale.

Once you are able to get a good referral and meet with your doctor, double down and ask questions to make sure your doctor is honest about their skill level and is willing to make decisions with you based on your goals. Again, easier said than done. Shannon Cohn advises, "When you go to the doctor's office, realize the power dynamic and try to change it, so that when you walk in, you look at your doctor as your partner, not as the be-all and end-all about your health. That's key. Don't just take whatever the doctor says as gospel. You're trying to find treatment. You're trying to find better care. You're trying to find a

What is your most embarassing/ funny/scary endo moment?

Going into one surgery where I was going to have a colonoscopy, laparoscopy, and hysteroscopy all during the same surgery. . . . I told my surgeons "they were going to be in all of my holes and to enjoy."

—Jillian Schurr

better way to take care of yourself together. If the doctor isn't being a good partner in that way and shuts you down or isn't listening to you, then I would say find another partner."

What Happens after Surgery?

Before or after surgery, you will most likely get a piece of paper with instructions on when you can return to work, drive, exercise, and go back to everyday life. Depending on the complexity of your surgery, the timing they suggest for returning to "normal" will vary. But from my own experience and countless other friendos I've spoken to over the years, the time line on that piece of paper is generally not generous enough.

You might feel great in the exact time they suggest. But you might not. Your appetite might be different. You might not want to be intimate or have your partner touch you (or even give you a hug, for that matter). You might feel more tired. Your periods might be different. Your bowel movements could be different, too. You just might not feel like yourself for a little while. And that's normal. That piece of paper is a general guideline and was most likely not tailored to your unique body. It also doesn't account for your stressors at home or work, the pressure you feel to bounce back, or any mental trauma you experienced having surgery. Shannon Cohn says, "How do you expect to be normal if you have been in intense physical and emotional pain for over a decade? Even if you have successful surgery, how would you expect your body to just rebound overnight? There's no way. You're going to have to help it a little bit to get it back to where it was."

Take it as slow as you can. Ask for help. And do your best to not judge yourself based on how long that piece of paper said it would take for you to be "normal" again. And if things don't feel right, do not feel any shame in contacting your doctor to say so.

After surgery, it's important to have your doctor thoroughly go over the surgery with you. Make sure to ask where they found and removed lesions and, most important, if they left any behind. This information is important. If you continue to suffer from painful bowel or urinary issues and you know that your doctor left lesions behind in those areas, then you'll know why. If you have had side pain for years, just knowing that your doctor removed lesions from your appendix can give you answers. Your doctor should also give you imagery taken during the surgery. If this is not provided to you, ask for it. This is something you should have access to.

And remember, no matter how good you feel after surgery, you must continue to get checkups. If you have a history of cysts, request to have an ultrasound every six months to once a year. I can tell you from firsthand experience, it matters. For five years, and over the course of seeing three different doctors, I asked if I could get an ultrasound referral at my annual exams. Even though I felt pretty good, I thought it was important to check in because I had a history of cysts. But all three doctors told me that I didn't need them because I wasn't in pain. My gut said to keep pressing, but after three doctors said no, I thought maybe I was being high-maintenance and stopped asking.

During this time, I grew a 10cm (3.94-inch) cyst that eventually ruptured and needed to be removed immediately. It was the most painful thing I have ever experienced in my life, and I thought I might not make it through the week leading up to my surgery. I know this pain and trauma could have been avoided if I had gotten the ultrasounds I requested. I vowed to never let that happen again. Now, when I meet with a new doctor, the first thing that comes out of my mouth is that I want to get an ultrasound referral every six months—and if they are not okay with that, then I won't be able to be their patient. I've yet to get a "no," and I have to say, I feel so empowered every time I get a "yes."

One final note about surgery: surgery alone might not be enough to manage your endo. You might be thinking, *Duh, that's why I bought this book.* Hear me out. So many of us think that surgery will solve everything. *If I could just have that operation, all my problems will be solved. My surgery will change my life!* And it might. Especially if you have lesions on sensitive areas or painful cysts. But it's also about what happens next. How will you complement and continue to nurture the progress that surgery provided? How will you make your care a priority? Can you continue to explore more options to support your health? The tools in this book are a great way to begin to do that, surgery or not. Even with the best surgery and all the tools in the world, you still might have bad days. But the hope is to have more good days than bad, and I want to try to help you achieve that in the pages ahead.

What about Hormonal Prescription Medications?

There is a lot of misinformation out there claiming that these medications are "treatments" for endometriosis, but they are not. They are designed to help manage pain and symptoms but not to treat the endometriosis itself. This is very important to understand and something that is often misrepresented.

Dr. Goldstein says these medications "can put your body in a menopausal state. It stops the hormonal stimulation of the lesion, but that doesn't guarantee that it stops the spread. We've had patients who, despite being on medications for ten years, have developed a bowel obstruction and required two or three bowel resections during those ten years." She says these medications are not magic, and they don't treat the disease the way excision does to stop endo in its place.

Dr. Goldstein does say that some patients do have relief taking these medications. But you must be mindful and aware of the side effects. They can cause bone loss, vaginal dryness, suicidal thoughts, and menopausal symptoms that many might not tolerate well, especially at a young age. The effects of long-term use of these medications have also not been evaluated. Make sure to keep track of how you feel while using them, and if you don't feel right, trust your gut and talk to your doctor right away.

If these medications are your doctor's first line of defense, and they're telling you they will stop your endo, ask more questions. Are they willing to talk about excision surgery and lifestyle-management tools, too? Are they able to discuss the side effects with you? What happens after taking these medications? What are the long-term effects of these drugs on your body? You have every right to ask these questions, and more. This is your body, not theirs. If they are unable to answer these questions and recommend these medications as your only option, consider getting a second opinion.

Do I Have to Be on the Birth Control Pill?

If you have endo, chances are your doctor probably told you that you *have* to be on the pill to manage your symptoms. But this is *your* choice, and similar to the medications we've talked about in this chapter, you need to be aware of the side effects and keep track of how they make you feel.

The pill is not a treatment for endo. Dr. Goldstein shares that it can help, because there is a suppressive effect on your ovaries and overall hormone system—and potentially on the bleeding/period itself. But it doesn't get rid of lesions, doesn't cure endometriosis, and most people will still have symptoms. Many people find relief on it and can take it to increase time between surgeries, or if they aren't able to afford surgery. But the jury is still out on whether the long-term use of birth control for endometriosis benefits outweigh the risks in terms of disease progression. In addition, Dr. Goldstein says that for some endo patients, their symptoms can break through the pill, meaning, "someone can use a pill for ten years and that works well, and then suddenly their symptoms can break through the pill's ability to suppress their symptoms."

There is also more research being done by women's health advocates about the concerns of the depressive and body-changing side effects of the birth control pill, including extreme mood shifts, suicidal thoughts, libido changes, and generally not feeling like themselves or in their own body while taking the pill. It becomes tricky for people who do find symptom relief from the pill yet feel the damaging mental effects.

Dr. Goldstein says that patients who suffer from severe anxiety, depression, or mental health issues (or if they're on medications for these) may not be the best candidates for the pill. If you are looking for alternative birth control methods, ask your doctor and do your own research for alternatives and their side effects.

To be clear, if the pill helps you and you feel good taking it, carry on! But I've heard too many stories over the years from friendos who were told that the pill can help them get rid of their endo (it can't) and/or they suffered from the damaging mental health effects of being on the pill. Ultimately, it's up to you to decide what's right for you, mentally and physically.

Which endo symptoms do you most despise?

On my worst days, the pelvic pain . . . makes it incredibly painful for me to stand. I keep chairs in my bathroom and chairs in my kitchen so I can sit while I do my makeup or brush my teeth, and while I cook. It can be really disabling.

—Jane Aldridge

If you want to dive deeper into this topic, *This Is Your Brain on Birth Control: The Surprising Science of Women, Hormones, and the Law of Unintended Consequences* by Sarah E. Hill, PhD, and *Beyond the Pill* by Dr. Jolene Brighten are incredible resources to learn more.

Is Getting a Hysterectomy a Cure for Endo?

No. But at the time of writing this, some of the top medical websites and institutions in the country still list "a hysterectomy" as a treatment for endometriosis. This is simply not true. Leslie, a friendo living in Oregon, shares that she was diagnosed with endo years *after* getting a hysterectomy for her pelvic pain. Dr. Goldstein backs this up. If there is still endometriosis disease left behind during the hysterectomy, and it is not excised, those endo implants can still cause pain and other issues.

But Dr. Goldstein also shares that for many people, a hysterectomy can help. If most of a patient's pain is central, related to uterine cramping, and the period itself, they may get relief from a hysterectomy. She says it's also important to note that for many patients with adenomyosis, this may be like a cure—they will never have a painful period again and may never need surgery again. But this is not to be misinterpreted as the "cure" or "end-all" for all endometriosis lesions, and it should never be seen as the first line of defense. All patients should remember that they always have a choice, and if they choose this path, it should include deep excision if possible of all visible disease.

More to Know

Does Endometriosis Only Affect Cisgender White Women?

No. But the media, and even medical institutions, have historically presented it that way. In fact, up until 2020, one of the top hospitals in the country shared on their website that "white women" had an increased risk of having endometriosis. There are no current studies to prove this. And it wasn't until Kyla Canzater, a women's health and endometriosis advocate, rallied to have this changed that it was removed from their website.

Kyla explains that that single line on the hospital's website was an example of the systemic problems in our healthcare system that must be changed. She said that when a person first experiences pain, they usually head to Google and look at hospital websites because the websites are believed to be credible. And when a person of color sees that "white women" are more prone to getting endometriosis, they might think, *Well, maybe I don't have endo*, and then they won't ask questions and/or press their doctor to explore it with them. So, they move on. Stay silent. Live with their pain. And in turn, this lengthens diagnosis times for people of color and can lead to fertility and self-esteem issues down the road.

Most of us are already familiar with the healthcare disparities between women and men in the United States, but add the layer of being a woman of color and the equity of care decreases even further. In a meta-analysis on how race and ethnicity play a role in how long it takes to receive an endometriosis diagnosis, Black and Hispanic women were nearly half as likely to be diagnosed with endometriosis as white women.[1]

Kyla says that, as a Black woman, she has always felt the need to be "overly educated" and "present [herself] in a certain way" in order for a doctor to take her seriously and get the care she needs. A 2016 study showed that nearly half of medical students and residents believed that Black patients felt less pain than white ones. Another showed that 29 percent of Black patients and 22 percent of Hispanics/Latinos were less likely to receive treatment with opioids than white patients with the same condition.[2]

————

In addition to the racial bias happening in our healthcare system, the LGBTQ+ and gender-nonconforming endo community faces huge disparities in access to proper care. A survey conducted by Lambda Legal revealed that "almost 56 percent of lesbian, gay or bisexual (LGB) respondents and 70 percent of transgender and gender-nonconforming respondents" had "experienced at least one of the following types of discrimination in care: being refused needed care; healthcare professionals refusing to touch them or using excessive precautions; healthcare professionals using harsh or abusive language; being blamed for their health status; or healthcare professionals being physically rough or abusive." At the time of writing this, a healthcare professional can choose to deny care to a transgender or gender-noncomforming patient for no reason other than their gender identity.

Alea, a friendo who identifies as queer, shares that she's definitely struggled with finding doctors to help her. In the past she had a shaved head, chose not to shave her armpits, and dressed in boy's clothes. And during this time, none of her doctors ever brought up pregnancy or fertility (the way they typically do with every other person with endo). "It's funny," she says, "because all I've ever wanted is to have kids. I can't wait to get pregnant." During a different encounter, a doctor told her that painful sex wouldn't apply to her because she was queer. She corrected the doctor and told her "queer people have all types of sex."

So, no. Endo is not a cisgender white woman's disease. And I want to end this section with a big hug and say how much better it's getting each day, but we still have a way to go in terms of equity in our health-care system.

How can we continue to push to make changes and support everyone in the endo community? Now that you know this is happening, learn more. Create awareness. Educate others in your community. Vote on these issues. Donate. Write letters. Ask your doctor what policies they have in place to provide equal care to their patients. People like Kyla and Alea are speaking up, and organizations like Endo Black and the Human Rights Campaign are helping foster change, but there needs to be more voices demanding it. Why not be one of them?

Is It Common for People with Endo to Have Other Health Conditions, Too?

Dr. Goldstein says people with endo have a higher risk of developing comorbidities (the presence of more than one condition) than those without. These conditions may include: overactive bladder, IC (interstitial cystitis, a painful bladder syndrome), irritable bowel syndrome, nickel sensitivity, celiac, menstrual migraines, anxiety and depression, sexual dysfunction, fibromyalgia, and other autoimmune diseases (including Sjögren's syndrome and Hashimoto's thyroiditis). There is also an increased risk of ovarian and other gynecological cancers.

Not everyone with endo will have additional health conditions, but it's important to understand the possibility that some of these conditions may occur. It's easy to blame everything on your endo, which means you could overlook something else at play. Dr. Goldstein says to remember that with multiple diseases, it takes a team approach to care, and she always recommends collaborating with your endo specialist and a thorough internist.

Why Do I Have a Lot of Bathroom Issues (Diarrhea and Bladder and GI Symptoms)?

One study has shown that 90 percent of people with endo have GI symptoms (bloating, constipation, diarrhea, gassiness),[3] which explains why so many people with endometriosis are diagnosed with IBS before getting an endo diagnosis. Dr. Goldstein explains that with endo, "you're more likely to have an inflammatory bowel system, and you're a bit more likely to be sensitive to things. The bowel and the bladder immediately surround the uterus. Frequently, they are involved because they are 'the next of kin.' When disease causes scar tissue and inflammation, it's going to cause problems for its neighbors as well. Oftentimes bowel symptoms can be a sign of endometriosis. It can cause serious GI irritation and other side effects." Many people with endo experience gut dysbiosis, SIBO (small intestinal bacterial overgrowth), and other GI conditions. So, it's important to be aware of your GI symptoms and track when these symptoms occur to help better inform yourself and your doctor of what's going on. Paying attention and tracking which of these symptoms are exacerbated with certain foods can give you critical information, too (something we'll be talking about more in the Good Food chapter ahead).

Why Am I So Bloated That I Look Pregnant?

See above. And in addition to GI symptoms, many people with endo can have inflammation of their appendix, colon, or the lining of the abdomen that can cause bloat and swelling.

Wearing looser-fitting pants and dresses (I love caftans) can help to deal with some of the pressure of an distended belly. But bodily discomfort may only be part of the problem. Sometimes your pregnant-looking belly, a.k.a. "endo belly," can alter the way you see yourself in the mirror and create body dysmorphic issues and/or weight obsession. And being asked if you're pregnant for the third time in one week because of your bloated belly can lead to having deep insecurities around wearing form-fitting clothes, especially bathing suits. One friendo shared that the pregnancy question is one of the cruelest questions for her. Because although she might look pregnant, she wasn't able to carry a child because of her endo-related fertility issues.

I wish there was a magic pill for this one, but unfortunately, no matter how well you take care of yourself, sometimes a bloated belly is out of your control. A low-inflammatory diet, tracking foods that make you more bloated, and practicing stress-management practices can help (more on all of this later in the book). Do your best to find clothes that make you feel comfortable. If you experience body-dysmorphic and weight-obsession issues, talk to a professional if you can. I also find it very comforting to have a handful of comebacks ready for whenever the "When are you due?" and pregnancy-related questions come at me, to shut the conversation down.

Feel free to steal one of these . . .

"No baby. Just a giant ovarian cyst!"

"I'm not pregnant. Are you?!"

"Nah, babies are gross."

Why Am I So Tired?

Endo fatigue is truly one of the hardest symptoms to manage. Because no matter how well you eat or how much you sleep, some days it feels like you drank twenty margaritas the night before *and* stayed up with a newborn baby. Endo fatigue is an intense, deep, and permeating feeling of exhaustion that can be hard to shake, no matter how hard you try.

Similar to an autoimmune disease, having endo means your body experiences a constant state of inflammation. Dr. Goldstein says the fatigue can be caused by "an overwhelming inflammation and immune response in your body that wears you down. It's not typically just the period or the ovulation itself but the systemic response recruiting immune help and factors around all these little lesions, similar to when your body is fighting a virus and attracting immune-system cells to help attack."

While we might not be able to always beat this fatigue, knowing why it happens can be helpful. You might not ever be able to knock it out completely, but for some, it is possible to help lessen the load with low-inflammatory foods, stress management, and movement practices (again, we'll be learning about these soon).

How Does Endometriosis Impact Fertility?

Remember that diagnosis-day scenario we ran through at the beginning of the chapter? On the day that most people with endo are diagnosed, the first thing they are told is to start thinking about getting pregnant (if they haven't already). This is problematic for many reasons. For starters, not every person wants or feels it necessary to have a biological child, and some do not want children at all. And if they do, not every person is in the position to have one, whether that be for financial reasons or not wanting to have a child on their own (if they do not have a partner).

Also, contrary to what many doctors say, getting pregnant is not a "treatment" for endo. Dr. Goldstein says, "Getting pregnant can suppress symptoms, because there will be a cessation [stopping] of your period for a year or longer with pregnancy. If you breastfeed, many people have suppression even longer and feel good with the high progesterone–balanced state it causes. But it does not make the disease itself go away."

But back to the question: Yes, endometriosis can affect fertility. Some people with endo can have a difficult time getting pregnant and carrying a baby full term, while others are able to have children with no issues. We don't always know why, but there are some factors that can play a role in this.

Here's what we do know. Dr. Goldstein shares that up to 50 percent of patients with unexplained infertility have endometriosis—potentially more if you consider that most of these people are not having a laparoscopy. Endometrioma in the ovary suppresses ovarian function. Inflammation plays a role, and the actual lesions themselves can cause a physical scar or problem with the fertility system. Transport from the fallopian tubes can be altered by adhesions—or the tube itself could be blocked from scarring. Endo can cause subfertility (reduced fertility) issues. Adenomyosis in the uterus can cause higher risk of fertility problems. And we also know that many people with endo have very painful sex, which can make trying to get pregnant naturally a traumatic and extremely difficult experience. But this isn't a "doomsday diagnosis," as Dr. Goldstein says. It is possible for many people with endometriosis to get pregnant.

Dr. Goldstein advises that if you do want a biological child, it's worth being proactive about your fertility. This could mean meeting with a fertility specialist, taking a fertility-hormone test, putting a management plan in place, and getting proper endometriosis treatment (more and more evidence shows that excision surgery can help increase the ability to conceive). Again, this might not be an option for all patients, but having a consultation with a specialist is a good start.

Dr. Goldstein also shares that if you're in your twenties, egg-freezing technology has come a long way over the years. It's an option that can give people better peace of mind and take the pressure off themselves, especially when dating. She says that she's hopeful that there will be insurance coverage one day for endo patients, because it does come with a price tag, but there are currently some financial-assistance programs for egg freezing out there.*

The topic of endo and fertility is complicated and vast—one that cannot be covered in a small section of this book. So, if you have more questions, I encourage you to speak to a specialist. Fertility issues are not just physically challenging but emotionally challenging, too. In the next chapter, we're going to talk more about the emotional aspects and about alternative paths to becoming a parent.

Will My Endo Go Away with Menopause?

Dr. Goldstein says that if you're perimenopausal, your periods might get worse before they get better (this can also happen in people without endo). But with endo, perimenopausal symptoms can be more intense, because during this time you generally have more frequent periods (every two weeks instead of every four). They may even be heavier first before going away.

Once you are in menopause, ovulatory pain should get better. Dr. Goldstein says most endometriosis patients will do much better with menopause because they have less hormonal stimulation. And some have complete relief. But if there are lesions in areas like the bowel, around the uterus, or around the bladder, those may still be symptomatic and continue to cause issues. While in perimenopause and menopause, it's still important to continue to use endo management tools, such as paying attention to diet, movement, and stress-management practices.

Why Am I Learning a Lot of This Information for the First Time?

I know. It's frustrating, and this can bring up a lot of emotions. Heather Guidone says, "By and large, endometriosis in and of itself has been

---

* In 2020, New York State passed a bill that insurance providers for large employers are required to cover some IVF and even egg freezing for patients with endometriosis. This is a huge step, which will hopefully be adopted in other states and by all employers.

ignored forever. The associated menstrual pain that many people with endometriosis have is dismissed or otherwise ignored. And there's this real legacy of stigma and inaccuracy that surrounds endo that's continually shared in perpetuity." But, she says, "it's changing as we speak."

It is changing.

There are advocates fighting for you, and there is more and more awareness and education of endo out there. Yes, it still might not be enough, but we're getting there and need to celebrate the progress that people like Dr. Goldstein, Shannon, Casey, and Heather have made for us already. And now *you* have this information to not only empower yourself, but to share, educate, and empower the next generation of people with endo.

Life with Endo

Every year on my birthday, I write down my goals and intentions for the coming year. No matter where I am or who I am with on that day, I seclude myself for an hour with no phone or distractions and really focus on what I want to work on. I grab whatever paper I can find (one year it was on a bunch of restaurant napkins, and another year it was some postcards I found at a gas station), then I break down my goals into three categories: 1. Relationships; 2. Personal (Mental/Physical Health); and 3. Career. I then start filling in each category. I always come back to these three categories or pillars, because over the years, I've discovered that if one is out of whack, the others tend to follow.

As I was starting to think about how to approach this chapter, my head was swirling with everything there is to say about living a life with endo, because sometimes it can feel like it impacts every single aspect of your day. I needed to organize those swirls, so I pulled out some sticky notes to break down the topics I wanted to cover. As soon as I grabbed a pen, without even thinking, I wrote down those three categories I write down each year. It was a little creepy (and cool) how my brain immediately went to them. After writing them out, I realized that these are the categories that living with endo impacts most.

As you work your way through each category, please think about how endo has impacted them for you. There will be some spaces where you can record these thoughts. I understand that some of the information and stories we'll be covering might hit close to home and bring up some emotions. Do your best to not judge yourself, your body, or how you might have acted in similar situations. Right now we're bringing more awareness to these pillars and how you might be able to work through them better in the future (or acknowledge and celebrate how great you're already doing). Let's jump in . . .

Relationships

For years my sister, Alissa, and I didn't get along very well. And I'm talking twenty-plus years. We got under each other's skin, and there were times we couldn't even be in the same room together. When we were younger, we fought with words and fists (and once there was an outright war with a plastic spoon from Dairy Queen). I'm embarrassed to admit it, but I was an aggressive, bratty, know-it-all older sister who loved to instigate drama. And Alissa was really angry and on edge most days, which only fueled the instigator in me. There were also some pretty big jealousy issues. Alissa was thin and an incredible athlete, whereas I was chubby and could barely run a lap around the school gym. Getting good grades and making friends came really easily for me, while Alissa struggled to do both at school. We wanted what the other had, and because of that, we found it really hard to find common ground. The one thing we did have in common was our pain. My sister has endometriosis, too. But because we rarely talked or got along, neither one of us knew just how much pain the other was in. I didn't even know Alissa had been diagnosed until years later through a conversation with my mom. Even after learning about her diagnosis, we went through cycles of hating each other and then almost liking each other, but then something would happen—and we'd start hating each other all over again. I didn't think it would ever be possible to have a healthy relationship with my sister.

But then it happened.

The same year I started to change my diet to manage my endo, Alissa did, too. During this time, we began to open up communication between us and send links to cookbooks that were helping us or articles we found supporting our new lifestyle. As Thanksgiving rolled around that year, we knew there wasn't going to be much that we could eat at our family's dinner, so we decided to hop on the phone (something we rarely did) and plan some dishes together. We had so much fun strategizing our Thanksgiving menu that I felt like I was talking to an old friend. Before we hung up, Alissa said something I'll never forget. She said, "I feel like this is our first Thanksgiving as sisters." I will always remember that moment, because things really changed for us after that call. We began to bond in a way that we never had before, and Alissa is now one of my closest friends. We text and talk all the time. Instead of being jealous of each other, we cheer each other on (she runs marathons now, and yes, I can still barely run a lap around the gym). We are able to reflect on our childhood and see all the things we did have in common back then. We are able to talk about endo and not feel so alone.

But the most important thing that we have in common now is that we're no longer in so much pain. We're both managing our endometriosis with the tools you're about to learn in this book. And now that we are each managing our pain, we can clearly see how most of our issues and anger toward each other was a result of that pain.

I don't ever want to use pain as an excuse for the way I've acted in the past. But I do acknowledge that pain played a role in our fractured relationship, because research shows that chronic illness and pain *can* affect our personalities, our moods, and how we connect with others.

Amber Murphy, a licensed psychotherapist and mental health coach who specializes in working with patients with chronic pain and women's issues (and has endo herself), shares that a lot of this is shaped in the time leading up to our diagnosis. "We don't understand what's happening in our body. We're being gaslit by doctors and the medical system. So, people start feeling unsafe in their bodies and unsafe in the world, and it starts shaping everything. Some people retreat and they go super internal and they withdraw. Other people, they lash out. Other people, their anxiety ramps up. It changes on an individual basis, but it can change every aspect of your personality. Just imagine if somebody walked around with an acute broken arm every day for the rest of their lives. Of course it's going to affect their personality, their mood, their patience, and their irritability level. There's just no way for it to not be impacted."

Amber explains that because we can't direct our anger at our endometriosis, we can begin to misdirect it. We start to project our anger, sadness, and feelings of hopelessness onto others. "We can feel so alone with these really big feelings that we end up displacing them and we tend to put them in safe places. For some people, that's road rage in the car, a safe bubble." For others, "it's our husbands, our wives, our partners, our parents—we tend to dump it in safe places where we know it can be received."

I don't think any of us want to hurt the people we love, and sometimes I'm not sure we're even aware that we're doing so. It becomes our norm to wake up feeling grouchy, sensitive, or irritable, and it's easy to take it out on the first person we see. Over time this can damage our relationships and, sadly, end some of them altogether. In an online survey I conducted with the Know Your Endo community, I asked, "What is the thing you struggle with most with endo?" One participant, Jen, shared that her biggest struggle was "not being able to maintain a social life. Constantly canceling plans or attempting to push through the pain and then being no fun to be around. I lost multiple friends because of this and ended up relocating across the country in hopes of a fresh start."

As someone who relocated a few years ago (though not because of endo), I can tell you that the old adage is true: "Wherever you go, there you are." Or in this case, "Wherever you go, your endo will follow." Yes, moving can give you an opportunity to create new relationships and a fresh start (and this might have been helpful for Jen). But even with new relationships, you cannot escape your endo. It's important to learn ways to communicate about your endo and create healthy relationships with those who are supporting you, and to find ways to communicate about your pain and let people know just what you're going through on a daily basis. I am not saying this will work with every person in your life. There will be some who may never understand, and these relationships will suffer. But we must at least try. And sharing how you feel doesn't have to be a big emotional reveal each time. Over time, it can become part of your everyday dialogue with family and friends.

So how do we begin to do this, *right now?*

Amber says "checking in" with your partner (or people close to you) before beginning to share is a good place to start. She gave this sample language to use: "Hey, I really want to share how I'm feeling with you right now. Are you in a place to receive it?" You can obviously change this language to fit your style. My style is yelling from my bedroom to my husband in the other room, "Hey! Can you come in here? I want to tell you about something. Is that cool?" *or* I'll send a simple text to a friend before I unload: "I'm struggling a little today. Got time to talk today or tomorrow?" Not as elegant as Amber's version, but these were huge first steps in being more mindful of how I share. After I do share, I always do my best to tell the person on the receiving end that if they're ever struggling, I'm there for them, too. It's a nice reminder that the caring and support does go both ways.

Amber understands that checking in isn't always possible, and it's a pretty high standard to practice all the time. But when we can, it's important to acknowledge that it can be hard for our loved ones, too. She explains, "It's hard to watch somebody that you love be in pain all the time and to be so helpless in it, to not be able to fix it, which I think is sometimes especially hard for men. It is hard to stand by somebody's side and watch them suffer and go through these difficult things and not be able to do anything to make it better."

Connecting and Dividing

Talking with Amber made me more curious to talk to partners and family members of people with endo to see how they cope. Out of all the conversations I had, the one that stuck out most was my talk with Greg, whose wife, April Christina, has endometriosis. Greg started our conversation by sharing that in the beginning of his relationship with April Christina, she initially didn't bring up her endo to him. But he did see her mention something about endometriosis on her social media, so he decided to "research it before she even had a chance to bring it up." He said he figured it must be important to her if she mentioned it and wanted to be ready (and admitted that he wanted to impress her a little, too).

When April Christina did bring up her endo, he was prepared with his notes. They talked about it, but he says she only gave him the introductory version and not the full picture of her pain. He told me, "There was a time when we were supposed to go on a date, and she was in the ER, and she didn't tell me until after. And then there's another time we were at her apartment and she couldn't move. It took everything in her body for her to move. She was reaching for some tissue, and I said, 'No, I'll get it. I'm already up.' And then she was like, 'No. No. I'll do it. I'll do it. I don't need your pity.' And I said, 'I'm not pitying you. I'm right here.' And then tears started to come down her eyes. I realized that it wasn't just about passing her the Kleenex."

Greg says that was a huge moment in their relationship, and he remembers telling her, "If we're going to be together, you're going to have to allow me to help you at times. We're going to have to learn how to balance it, because you can't try to do this on your own. At first, you had to do it on your own because you didn't have a choice, but now that you have help, don't refuse the help just because you want to prove something to yourself. You've already proven it."

Listening to Greg, it was clear that he's an incredibly supportive partner, but what does that support look like for the long haul? Did he ever get fatigued thinking about caring for someone who might experience pain and symptoms every single month, year after year? He says, "Help is not the issue. I think it's the balance of when to help and when not to help. I think that's where I get the fatigue. There are all kinds of moments where you may be limited, but you do what you can because you love the person. And you love the person more than you get frustrated with the illness. I made a promise to her. I said, 'Look. You don't have endo alone. We have endo. It affects both of us now. We both have to live with this. It's not only you anymore.'"

Greg has made a commitment to help his wife with whatever endo might bring, but unfortunately, this isn't always the norm. Over the years, I've received dozens of messages from people sharing how alone they feel because the people closest to them are not supportive. Yes, it hurts and feels frustrating to have your pain and symptoms dismissed by doctors and the healthcare system—but being dismissed by your family and friends can feel truly devastating, whether that's not believing your pain, getting upset when you cancel plans, or not being supportive of your choices to try to feel better. Margot, a friendo, says she battled with these issues. It's been a long road for her family to understand how endo has impacted her life.

Margot says that when she started having sex in college, she suffered from extreme pain that left her in bed for days. After a trip to the ob-gyn, her doctor said she probably had endo and that there was nothing else she could do about it and put her on the pill. Margot went on and off the pill for the next seven years, but she became increasingly depressed and her pain became unbearable. Still without a true diagnosis, she started researching and found holistic management tools that she thought might help her. She decided to take a chance on changing her diet to see if it could manage her symptoms. And it did. Changing her diet made a dramatic change in Margot's life, but her family wasn't totally on board with the changes she was making. She shared, "It was a very sore subject with my family for two years when I changed my diet." They told her she was being "difficult" and "too much" when she didn't want to eat certain things.

From talking to Margot, it was clear that her family loved her very much, but there was a divide between them when it came to the choices she was making to manage her health. Margot told me that she never doubted that her family didn't believe she had endo, but they just didn't take it seriously. They thought she was being "high-maintenance" and "dramatic." But when she was finally diagnosed and her family understood the extent of her disease, everything changed.

She remembers her mom and sisters crying after hearing her diagnosis from the doctor. They told her they didn't realize that everything she had been telling them all those years was as bad as it was. For the next three months after her diagnosis, Margot's mom brought it up all the time and felt tremendous guilt for not believing her. It was something they had to work through together as a family.

It's been a couple of years since her diagnosis, and Margot says her relationship with her family is "much better" now. Her mom makes recipes to support her diet and says her "sisters are definitely on board now." If Margot is feeling fatigued or not up for leaving the house, they respect it way more than they did in the past. They allow her to take the time she needs to feel better.

For Margot, it took her family hearing her diagnosis from a doctor to understand the severity of her condition. For others, it's taken ER visits, counseling, and, sadly, the loss of a pregnancy for them to find more empathy. When I see or hear of people struggling to find support from family and friends, my first instinct is to get mad for them and tell them to get that partner, friend, or family member out of their life. But it's not always that simple, and it may be a pretty unfair response. Relationships are complicated, and unless you're in it, you will never know the full picture. Just because someone doesn't understand your condition doesn't mean they don't love you or want to support you. Sometimes they don't know how to. While I don't think it's our sole responsibility to educate our loved ones about endo (hello, internet), sometimes we can gently nudge people in the right direction. Sometimes it takes meeting them where they are and giving them a crash course in Endo 101.

This could mean watching the endometriosis documentary *Endo What?* together or sending links to medical journals or printing out articles you've found online. You could take your partner/parent/friend to a doctor's appointment. Or show your surgery photos as a visual to help someone understand how endo has impacted different parts of your body and how it's not just a bad period. You could also bring a friend or family member to an endometriosis event to hear experts speak on the topic and give them an opportunity to talk to other people supporting those with endo. Sometimes if I'm really struggling for someone to "get it," I'll share that, in more severe cases, endometriosis lesions have spread to people's lungs. This always wakes up the person I'm talking to because they would likely be scared out of their minds if something was growing on *their* lungs.

While it can be helpful to find ways to better communicate about your endo, it's also important to continue to put your mental and physical health first. If you feel unsafe, unsupported, or if someone in your life is making you feel worse, it might be necessary to reevaluate those relationships.

Irene, a friendo in Amsterdam, did just that. She shares that everything was great with her boyfriend until she started experiencing a lot of endo symptoms. She started wearing loose dresses because of her endo belly, and her boyfriend would criticize her clothes and try to control what she wore. He began to criticize other aspects of her life, too. He continued to put her down, and Irene began to accept it as her new normal because she thought her "illness was difficult for him" and she just wasn't a "fun girlfriend." Irene says she felt like she was a burden and adopted an attitude of "I'm sorry I'm here" and "I'm sorry I'm taking up space." Whenever her boyfriend was around, Irene became tense waiting for him to criticize her. She became so tense that she couldn't be intimate with him anymore because it hurt too much. She thought sex was a part of her life that she'd have to say goodbye to forever. Things escalated, and Irene made the decision to leave her boyfriend. When she did, she realized something big: "I blamed everything on endometriosis and didn't realize he was just a shit guy."

Since ending her relationship, Irene said she still experiences pain, but it's so much less because she can actually relax now. She said it feels "like a miracle" how much better her symptoms are since moving out. She understands that being so tense all the time was contributing to her pelvic pain (we'll discuss the impact stress has on our bodies and endo in Chapter 5). Irene is even able to have sex again, something she thought she would never be able to do. She's now in a relationship with a partner who supports her. At first, she was surprised and would be overly grateful when her new boyfriend would ask her if she needed something when she was in pain. She said that he had to remind her that being nice to your partner is actually "normal relationship stuff."

All relationships are wildly different, and some can be rather complicated. You know best how the people in your life make you feel. But it is important to take a look at how your relationships are affecting you and your endometriosis. To have the conversations (even if difficult) to get the support you need. And in some cases, letting go of your pride and *accepting* the help that people want to give you.

And What about Parenting with Endo?

There are times when it feels too hard to get yourself ready for the day, let alone help someone else. You can't call in sick as a parent, and there are moments when you simply do not have a choice to not push through, no matter how much you want to climb back in bed. Unless you have the means to hire a chef, a couple of nannies, and a car service, it's on you to care for your children, no matter how bad you feel. Yes, many people with endo have supportive partners to help, but there are also a lot of solo parents out there with endo who don't have a support system. Ultimately, you just have to do your best, and that is why making your endo care a priority is critical.

As parents, we often feel guilty putting ourselves first. But I can tell you that I'm a 100 percent better parent because of the tools in this book and designating the time I need to take care of me. That time doesn't necessarily mean hour-long, candlelit bubble baths. It's little things like letting my son watch a show so I can get twenty minutes to move my body. It might mean ordering a meal-delivery kit on the first two days of my period to take the pressure off of cooking. And sometimes it means "going to the bathroom," which actually means sitting in an empty tub for ten minutes with my eyes closed or reading a chapter of a book. I never feel guilty about doing any of these things, because I know I'll be a kinder and more engaged parent after allowing myself to do them.

Louise, a friendo living in York, England, who is a mother of five and works part-time, shares, "Parenting is hard work as it is, never mind when you have a chronic health condition." She says that she really struggled with the physicality of it all when her children were younger: giving them baths, playing with them, and carrying them around. She also had less patience because of her pain, which didn't feel fair. But now that they are older and more independent, things have gotten easier, and she shared that "one of the most valuable things I've learned as a parent on my endo journey is to be as open as possible about the condition, so they understand it." Louise says that some days her kids can just tell by looking at her that she isn't feeling so great, so they rally and help her around the house.

Louise told me that endo has "become a part of their life like it has mine. Not always in a negative way, either." She explains that over the last year she has made significant changes to her eating and exercise habits that have transformed her life. "The children have now seen that even when you're diagnosed with a condition, you can turn it into a positive. You can take action and take back control, and I think that's a very valuable life lesson for them and it's also impacted family life positively. The change in my health has been so drastically different, and they often refer to it as an example of how you can turn a negative into a positive."

Louise's story is yet another example of how taking care of you can help you take better care of the people you love around you.

Sex*

Irene was able to relax enough to have sex again. But for some people with endo, even if you're relaxed and have the greatest and most supportive partner ever, sex can be extremely painful. Not just painful in the moment, but in the hours, and even days, after having sex. Painful sex is one the most predominant symptoms of endometriosis, but it's also one of the hardest to talk about.

Whether you learned about sex from an older sibling or from a class in high school, it came with the assumption that it's something we can all do, pain-free. We're told that the "first time" might hurt a little, but

---

* *We're talking about penetrative sex here. But it's important to note that some people with endo also suffer from vulvodynia, a chronic pain condition that occurs in the vulva (the area outside of your genitals) that causes feelings of burning, itching, and stinging. It's important to speak to your doctor if you're experiencing this pain.*

after that it's magical, it connects us to our partners, and it's fun! We hear about our friends having amazing sex, and watch movies with couples having wild and uninhibited sex, again all pain-free. So it's understandable how confusing and shameful it can feel when this is not your experience.

Some experience painful sex, but for others, sex and intimacy get more complicated because of fatigue, cramping, a bloated belly, and the fear and/or embarrassment of someone seeing their surgery scars. Whether it's pain alone or a combination of all of the above, these feelings are completely normal to have, but over time they can be extremely damaging. Studies show that painful sex (and avoidance of intimacy) because of endometriosis can result in lower self-esteem and feelings of guilt and inadequacy.[1] And all of this is in addition to causing tension in our relationships.

This is why communication is key. We need to have open and honest conversations to help our partners understand our bodies better and figure out ways to have sex that are enjoyable for *everyone* involved. These conversations are so important because it can be really hard during the act to ask our partners to stop because of pain. We don't want to make them feel bad for hurting us or be the reason they don't get to enjoy something that makes *them* feel good. It can feel just as hard to admit that you're "not in the mood" because of a bloated belly or other endo-related symptoms. We never want to put our partners in the position of feeling rejected. And because all of this is so hard, we often don't speak up and simply endure the mental and physical pain and suffer the consequences, during and after.

I'm not saying these conversations are ever easy. And I'm not suggesting you need to bring these things up on a first date or put it in your dating profile ("I'm an account manager who loves to travel, am obsessed with Italian food, and am prone to really painful sex!"), but it is important to figure out ways to talk about it. Put yourself on the other side for a second. Wouldn't you want to know if your partner was in pain? Wouldn't you want to know the reason why your partner avoided intimacy with you? Wouldn't you want them to enjoy sex right along with you?

This communication isn't just for new relationships, either. We all need to have these conversations, whether we've been with a partner for six months or six years. In the early years of my relationship with my now husband, I would often endure horrific pain during sex and then go to the bathroom afterward and cry. When I returned to bed, he had no idea of the pain I experienced. He'd want to lie together and cuddle. But instead of feeling happy in his arms, I'd lay there feeling uneasy and anxious because I felt like I was deceiving him. He had no idea he was hurting me, and I knew it would break his heart if he knew, so I kept it a secret. But over time, I couldn't continue lying to him, so I started sharing. A huge weight was lifted once I was able to share, and it actually brought us closer together.

Sharing doesn't have to mean big, formal, sit-down discussions. When you're having sex, you can experiment with new positions and find alternatives to intercourse. Dr. Uchenna Ossai, a pelvic health therapist, explains, "Penetration is not the gold standard" of sex. If you have painful sex or issues with intimacy because of your endo, she suggests trying pleasure mapping with yourself or with a partner. Pleasure mapping is exploring and discovering the parts of your body that you feel pleasure from (and ones that you don't) outside of your genitals. This could be the inside of your thigh, neck, breasts, or parts you never thought about. Dr. Ossai also says it's important to feel safe and secure before you sensitize this to sexual pleasure. Doing this can help you and/or your partner find ways to enjoy being intimate without the pressure to have intercourse.

You can also track which times of the month hurt most, so you're able to be more prepared. You can bring in different tools like lube and/or penis buffers that can control the deepness of penetration (Ohnut makes a great one). And I'm all about body positivity, but it is perfectly acceptable if you don't love your body every single day because of your bloat or scars. Wear (or don't wear) things that make your body more comfortable. Do it with super-dim lighting or no lights at all, if that makes you feel better. A friendo of mine takes a little cannabis before sex to help her body relax. Remember: it doesn't matter what everyone else is doing or how positive they are about *their* bodies. Just do what works for *you* so you can enjoy sex, too.

It's not just our partners we need to speak to. We need to communicate with our doctors, too. Talking with your doctor might help them better determine where your endometriosis lesions are located and/or help you find a treatment and management plan for pain with a specialist.

Heather Jeffcoat, a physical therapist and the author of *Sex without Pain: A Self-Treatment Guide to the Sex Life You Deserve*, specializes in helping people have pain-free sex. She says, "The majority of my patients who have endometriosis don't just have sexual dysfunction. A lot of them also have painful bladder syndrome, urinary urgency and frequency, or bowel dysfunction." She continues, "I really have to understand their whole pain process, not just related to sexual function, really understanding the timing of things, like how long does it hurt and what's the intensity. Because, as I explain to every patient, it's extremely important to be able to measure those changes." She says that short-term goals are important. "Let's say putting in a tampon is painful, as well as intercourse, but there's obviously a big difference between a tampon and intercourse. One early goal might be that they're able to insert a tampon pain-free or take a tampon out pain-free," and then work with dilators to gradually be able to tolerate more. Heather says intravaginal massage and neuromuscular stretching techniques can help, too. If people are really struggling with the intimacy aspect, especially if they can't have penetrative sex, Heather often gets a sex therapist involved to help her patients work through their mental and emotional issues.

But in some cases, even if you work with a specialist like Heather or try every position out there, sex still might hurt. Heather says, "With endometriosis, it's more complicated." Depending on where the endometriosis lesions are located, it can still be painful, "and I can't remove the endometriosis through pelvic physical therapy. Only surgery can excise that and remove the endometriosis." And research shows that removing endometriosis through excision surgery has helped patients with painful sex symptoms and improved their sex lives.[2] Excision surgery, of course, is not always an option for everyone. But I do like to share it, because someday soon, I hope it will be a more viable solution for everyone.

Now You.

How has endo impacted your relationships or sex life?

_____

_____

_____

_____

_____

_____

_____

What ways can you better communicate or accept help when it's being offered to you?

_____

_____

_____

_____

_____

_____

_____

Who are the people in your life who make you feel better and/or
worse when you are going through hard times with your endo?

_____

_____

_____

_____

_____

_____

Personal (Mental + Physical) Health

In 2019, the BBC conducted a survey with over 13,500 women on the
impact that endo had on their lives.[3] Nearly every person who contributed to the study said that endo had a negative impact on their mental
health. And almost half said they had suicidal thoughts because of endo
(and the majority used prescription painkillers to cope). While these
statistics are heartbreaking and shocking, they're not surprising. Living with a chronic illness can have a detrimental effect on our mental
health and cause psychiatric disorders, most notably anxiety and depression.* While depression is not a symptom of endo, for many it feels
like a by-product of the condition. In fact, it's been shown that people
with endometriosis have an elevated risk of developing depression and
anxiety disorders because of their condition, in addition to phobic anxieties and sensitivity being higher in patients with endometriosis than
those without.[4,5]

Amber Murphy, the psychotherapist we heard from earlier in this

---

* _It's important to note that you can be pain-free but still experience the
emotional impact of living with endometriosis._

chapter, says it's almost impossible "to go through the experience of not understanding what's happening in your body, not getting good answers from doctors, and not come out of that without some sort of trauma or anxiety and/or depression."

One of the trickiest parts about this experience is being able to separate your endo from your mental-health issues, especially if you've had a history of depression or any psychological disorders. *Is my fatigue a result of my endo, or am I depressed? Or am I depressed because of my endo and that depression is causing me to experience more fatigue? But also, I heard birth control can cause depression in some people, so is it the birth control that's making me sad? But also, I am supposed to be taking birth control to manage my endo, so should I stop?* The questions feel endless and can often spiral out of control.

The spiral can lead to pain catastrophizing, flooding your mind with negative and catastrophic responses to anticipated pain or pain that is actually happening. Catastrophizing has been shown to increase depression, and in people with chronic conditions, this can lead to feelings of hopelessness and the inability to shift your attention away from your negative thoughts to cope with the pain itself.[6,7]

Here's an example: In the morning, you feel a small cramp on your side. The catastrophic thinking turns on, and your mind tells you that this small cramp will surely turn into bigger and more painful cramps as the day goes on. Those cramps will become so bad that you'll have to miss your best friend's birthday party that night. You tell yourself that your best friend will be really annoyed about you missing another event and will have finally reached her limit on your serial canceling. You imagine all your friends at the party asking why you're not there, and they'll all roll their eyes when they find out you're "sick" again. Pretty soon, no one will want to hang out with you. Why would they want to? You can't even show up to your best friend's birthday party. Within minutes, your mind has created an outcome where you have no friends because of a small cramp.

When someone else who does not have a history of pain gets that same small cramp, they might think it's a little gas or a result of working out too hard the day before. They think, *That's strange*, and assume it will go away. Their brain doesn't go to the pain-catastrophizing mode. Their brain moves on. But when you've experienced pain for years, it's hard to do that. Amber says, "The best predictor for future pain is past pain." Maybe you've had a small cramp that turned into an emergency room visit and a ruptured cyst. Maybe a small cramp turned into a painful miscarriage. Maybe a small cramp turned into the worst period of your life and no one believed your pain. It's not your fault for the way your brain goes down this negative path. In some ways, it's trying to protect you and prepare you for what could happen. The problem with doing this is that catastrophizing pain can actually make your pain worse.

I want to be clear—this is not to say that your initial pain is not real. If you have pain, I believe you. As we know, endometriosis can be an incredibly painful condition. But in order to help manage your pain, you need to understand how to address it. Consistently check in with your mental health. Really check in. Working on your mental health with endo is just as important as your physical health. You can start doing that by becoming more aware of your catastrophizing patterns, seeking help from a therapist or endo support group, and, most important, creating coping tools to help your brain calm your body down (I'm excited to teach you about some in our stress-management week in Chapter 5).

Infertility + Creating Family in New Ways

As we learned in the previous chapter, having endometriosis doesn't mean that you are destined to have infertility or subfertility issues. But for those who do, the emotional toll can be significant, and it's often underplayed. I'm not sure we give enough weight to the suffering that the endo community experiences with these issues. We see the statistics, but it's rare that we hear the experiences of the people behind those numbers—people who are carrying a lot of grief, shame, and feelings of failure due to infertility.

In a survey I conducted with the Know Your Endo community, I asked how infertility—or the fear of it—has affected them, and here are some of their answers:

The mental devastation of infertility is so much more painful than the mind-blowing pain of period cramps, bloating, and sickness. Changing my diet and exercising more won't mean that I can conceive. It's the cruelest endo symptom I experience and the most difficult to talk about. —SW

Feeling less of a woman. Not good enough. Don't understand why my husband still sticks by my side when I can't give him children but also grateful for him. Constantly depressed but have to pretend to the world you are okay. Creating a shield/wall to protect yourself from everyone around you who reminds you that "you are not getting any younger" or "look at your younger sister with children, what are you waiting for?" Sometimes feeling like you hate your life and wish things were different. Crying myself to sleep at night. Praying to God but losing faith as everyone around you easily gets pregnant except you. Shutting out your friends unintentionally because you feel like you no longer have anything in common and you feel left out. Binge eating to drown away my sorrows. —CS

IVF was rather traumatic, as was finding out the risk to my health outweighed the chance of success, and that's not great motivation to keep going with this invasive procedure. —MG

It's definitely affected my confidence with dating. Deep down I know that if that bothered someone, they're not the one for me anyway. Everyone has their "baggage," and I do have a lot to offer, but it has been a huge mental block in moving forward in that area of my life in particular. It's been difficult emotionally to see friends around me who are starting to get engaged, pregnant, married, etc. Although I am grateful to have been diagnosed, it has been a difficult age to be going through it all, when so many of those around me are reaching milestones that I always thought I would be nearing alongside them. —ER

These women are not alone in their experiences. Fertility issues have been shown to cause depression, anxiety, loss of self-esteem, feelings of hopelessness, and grief.

Amber Murphy says, "There is a ton of grief" when you are not able to create a family the way you thought you would. She says, "The first step before you do anything is just sitting with the grief. Letting yourself have that without judgment." We must make space for it, "because people with endo are so constantly in survival mode, keeping our heads down and pushing forward, that sometimes we don't make space for ourselves to experience what's happening." She recommends working with a therapist if you can or talking to other people who have struggled with infertility. "It is really painful, and I think it's too much to be alone in. I don't know that our partners can necessarily understand in the same way." And oftentimes our friends and family who haven't experienced these issues won't understand, either.

Dr. Goldstein, who you heard from in the previous chapter, shares that she struggled for years to have a child because of endo. She went through multiple rounds of IVF, and during that time, her family and friends kept telling her that once she had a baby, she wouldn't even remember all she went through to get there. But she told me that even now that she has a healthy baby girl, she'll never forget. She won't ever

What have you lost because of your endo?

Relationships, careers, fertility, normality—other than that it's been fine! I haven't lost my sense of humor and I haven't lost those I love most in the world—that's what I remember at my lowest.

—Eleanor Thom

forget the grief and struggles she experienced trying to conceive and what it took to create her family (and makes her grateful for each moment).

It's important to remember that it's okay if you aren't able to "just move on" or want to yell at the well-meaning person who tells you "everything happens for a reason" for the umpteenth time. It is a real loss to lose a child through miscarriage. It is a real loss not to create your family the way you'd dreamed. It is a real loss to discover you cannot carry a child. These losses are significant, and you need to give yourself space to grieve and process them.

Amber says that once you're able to process your grief, it's about "moving on to solutions, not rushing toward solutions." If you do decide that you want to create your family in an alternative way, she says, "It's really important not to rush that process and to give ourselves time within that process," and that each of our paths might be different and that's okay.

Navigating a Different Path

If you do decide to create your family through adoption, foster-to-adopt, surrogacy, or egg donation, it's important to find and talk with families who have gone through the process before. There is a lot of misinformation out there about these "alternative ways" to create your family, and the media doesn't help by focusing on the worst-case-scenario stories.

Talking to other families who have been through it will give you a fuller picture of the process, the obstacles they've faced, and the things they wished they would have known before starting. You'll also get to hear the joy they felt when they met their child for the first time, too.

It's important to have these conversations and hear real-life, positive stories and not only rely on the sensationalized versions, a.k.a. Lifetime movies, for this information.

Because of the misinformation and lack of positive stories/outcomes out there, you might find that your family and friends don't understand the process you're going through to create your family, and they may be critical and/or have a lot of questions about your decision. *Aren't you scared what kind of baby you're going to get? What if the birth mom decides to keep the baby? Isn't that super expensive? Are you worried about whether you'll be able to love the baby as your own?* You might be thinking that these questions seem a little invasive and inconsiderate (they are), but these are all very real questions I was asked when I chose to create my family in a way that made some people in my life feel uncomfortable.

I knew from a young age that I didn't want pregnancy for my body. Maybe I had endo angels who knew something about my fertility that I didn't and planted this seed in my young mind. I'm not sure. I just always knew that I wanted to create a family in a "different" way, and so that's what I did. I never tried to get pregnant and have never once regretted that decision. I hear more and more often from people with endo who say they don't want pregnancy for their bodies, either. They've already had so much trauma and pain in that area of their body, and they really aren't interested in having more. Even when you are confident that adoption, foster-to-adopt, or surrogacy is your first choice for creating your family, you still might be faced with judgment from others. *Are you doing this because you don't want to get fat during pregnancy? Are you secretly scared you can't get pregnant, so you don't want to try? Is there something wrong with your husband's sperm?* Again, these are actual questions I was asked! It baffled me why people cared so much about this very personal decision I was making. And this decision was my first choice to create my family. I can't imagine how devastating these questions are for the people who suffered from years of infertility to get to there.

People will most likely ask questions like these, so it's good to be prepared with responses for them. Depending on your mood or the person asking these questions, you can choose a couple of different routes. The first is a response that shuts it down immediately by saying, *This isn't something I feel comfortable talking about right now* or flipping it back to them with a *How's YOUR husband's sperm?* or *Were you worried what kind of baby YOU were going to get when you gave birth?* You can also choose a response that's an opportunity to shine a positive light on different ways to create families. By educating the person asking the question, you can help them understand your decision, the overall process, and why that question could be hurtful (and hopefully they'll never ask it again to someone else).

I have to tell you that writing about the topic of infertility is one of the most challenging endeavors I've faced writing this book. I can't say anything that will make the grief, struggles you may have faced, and/or loss go away. It's complicated, raw, and full of so many different emotions. What I can say is that if you are struggling, my hope is that you will reach out to someone to talk about it—a therapist, a friend, a friend of a friend who has gone through it, too. You do not have to carry this burden alone, and there are a lot of people out there who can and want to help you.

Now You.

How has endo impacted your mental health and/or perception of yourself?

_____

_____

_____

_____

Do you have an example of a time you have catastrophized your pain?

_____

_____

_____

_____

_____

Are there ways that you can be kinder to yourself or get help to have better mental health with endo?

_____

_____

_____

_____

_____

_____

_____

Work

Over the last twenty-five years I've had a lot of jobs. I've been a gas station attendant. I've made pizzas, wedding cakes, and Blizzards at Dairy Queen. I've waitressed. I was a telemarketer. I owned a stationery brand and a bar (at the same time). I was a shopgirl at a hat store, and I was real estate agent's assistant (also at the same time). I creative-directed a clothing line. I worked for magazines and event companies . . . this list goes on and on. The jobs I've had over the years are pretty diverse, but there's one thing they've all had in common: I worked all of them, at one point or another, in debilitating pain.

Before I knew how to manage my endo (and before I knew I had endo at all), I was way too proud to ask for days off. I was determined to never let anyone see me sweat, or show an ounce of weakness. If I did call in sick or complain that I was in pain, I thought people might question if I was the right person for the job. They would see that I wasn't competent or reliable and find someone to replace me. And I couldn't risk that. I *needed* the money. I had rent, student loans, and bills to pay. Even with my own businesses, when the only person I reported to was *me*, I still dragged myself to work on my most painful days. I had employees to manage and was determined to never show any signs of weakness to them, either.

I remember those painful days like it was yesterday. Taking the train to work in so much pain that I thought I might pass out before I reached my stop. I wondered: *If I did pass out, would someone call 911 for me? Would they notify my husband? Should I hold my driver's license in my hand so they can easily identify me?* While everyone else around me was casually reading the newspaper or playing on their phones, I was planning how to make the paramedics' jobs easier when they found me.

When I finally did make it to work safe and sound, I would use the bathroom every hour or so to change my blood-soaked pad and/or deal with my GI issues. I'd have so much anxiety that someone might come in after me and smell all the things that my body was doing that I'd always try to choose the stall farthest from the door. When I wasn't in the bathroom, I'd be sitting at my desk just staring at my computer screen, not even able to think because of my fatigue. I remember feeling like there was no way I could sustain this for the rest of my life. But I *still* never took a day off.

I'm not alone in pushing through my pain and symptoms during all those years. Unfortunately, people with endometriosis have gotten really good at this. In a study conducted with over five hundred women with endometriosis in three different countries over the course of a month, 78.1 percent reported they took no sick leave. None. These women used their vacation time to recharge and even limited their free time outside of work to reserve their energy for their jobs.[8]

Victoria Williams, a researcher who focuses her work on endometriosis in the workplace, explains that people with endo "are suffering in silence to protect their job, promotions, and their credibility and reputation. When symptoms are at their worst—whether it's extreme fatigue, side effects of medication, menstrual bleeding, crippling pelvic pain—women with endometriosis will lose an average of around seven to ten hours per week of productivity." Victoria compared endo to working a third shift—"you're not just working in full-time employment, you're not just doing that second shift [the domestic work at home or maintaining a social life], but you're also managing a full-time illness that fluctuates constantly."

Being forced to work this third shift has affected the career trajectory of many people diagnosed with endo. It's been shown that people with endo have a lower likelihood of working in their desired profession and have a greater chance of being unemployed because of their condition.[9] Many decide to change jobs, take a pay cut, or choose part-time work because it's the only way to be able to make money while also managing their condition. Victoria shared that people with endo are "being discriminated against in the workplace, they're having to give up their chosen career, or they're having to give up full-time employment completely. And that obviously has an effect on your psychological well-being, if you're at home or you're not feeling as if you can participate in society."

Endo on the Job

Sabrina, a friendo living in New York, made the difficult decision to change jobs, due largely in part to her endo. Sabrina worked as a journalist and news producer for over a decade, which she says was a pretty high-stress career. "You go, go, go, rush, rush, rush, to get something on air, and every other hour you're running downstairs to the control room to make sure everything is going to be on air properly. It was a high-stress environment at times, and it was addictive. You're addicted to looking at your phone, watching the news, and making sure you're on top of everything. It's this constant adrenaline rush, because you get addicted to that fast-paced style and environment." But after struggling with years of infertility and being diagnosed with endometriosis at thirty-eight years old, she started to question her priorities and career path.

The decision to change jobs wasn't an easy one for Sabrina, and it didn't happen overnight. "It was years of realizing how uncomfortable I was and how uncertain I was. When it gets to the point that you can't really perform in your job as well as you would like to, that's a breaking point that you need to try to figure out." She told me that she was just not able to live the life she wanted to live when she was constantly beating her body down. Changing jobs helped her put more time into managing her health. Sabrina says her new job can be high-stress at times, but it's a "different kind of stress," because she's now able to have more flexibility to focus on managing her endo. I asked Sabrina if she missed her old career, and she said, "I miss journalism itself and that pursuit of truth, reporting, and storytelling," but she also said that she's "been able to translate all of that passion for storytelling and content creation and creativity" into the work she does now and the trade-off is worth it. "I think for a lot of people that have these pipe dreams growing up in America, it's hard to give up on those dreams. But it's also great to be able to adapt our dreams to the path and the way our life unfolds—to find and create new dreams."

While Sabrina was able to find a new job to suit her lifestyle with endo, others are finding ways to adapt their current lifestyle to suit their jobs. Katie, a truck driver in England, has made big lifestyle adjustments to help manage her endo while driving her sometimes twelve-hour shifts.

When Katie started researching endometriosis and saw how much inflammation played a role in it, she decided to gradually decrease the inflammatory foods she ate, and it helped her a lot. This meant getting really diligent about packing her own food each week and limiting the daily "sandwiches, crisps, and chocolate" she was typically eating while she drove. She explains that it was really hard to find healthy food on the road, let alone a parking spot to get it. And at some of the construction sites she delivered to, "you'd be lucky if there was a toilet, never mind anywhere to make a cup of tea." She now plans her meals for the week every Sunday and has really started to love cooking. Not only does her body feel better with her new foods, but she says planning ahead helps reduce her stress, and she's saved a lot of money, too. Katie also makes sure to move her body more because she is sitting so much during her shifts. When she makes her deliveries, she'll make a point to get out of her truck and walk around. She started doing yoga, and the day I interviewed her, she shared that she had tried Pilates for the first time (and liked it).

Talking with Katie and hearing her positivity and dedication to managing her endo was truly remarkable. I wondered if she ever gets frustrated or down about the need to plan ahead. She says, "Sometimes." But she also says she always tries to look at the bigger picture. "Before I was quite disassociated or unattached

What is your most embarrassing/funny/ scary endo moment?

Last year, at the age of thirty-eight, I had my first symptomless period. I experienced none of the telltale signs: no mood change, no cramps, no hunger. I walked joyously into the makeup trailer at work, a trailer full of women, and asked if anyone had ever had such a wondrous thing happen to them. They all shrugged: "All the time." I didn't realize that a completely pain-free period even existed.

—Mozhan Marnò

from my body, I suppose. . . . I feel a lot stronger now, and I know my own boundaries, but I've also tried so many new things because I've had to kind of look outside the box a little bit. I think I live a much better life, and I feel better in myself now anyway despite having endometriosis. In a way it's kind of a blessing in disguise a little bit, you know?"

Creating New Standards

As you've probably gathered at this point, I love sharing endo success stories like Sabrina's and Katie's. But for as many endo work success stories as there are, I know there are just as many people struggling in the workplace. Victoria says we need menstrual policies in place to help those who are struggling: "We need to set a new standard for female needs. So that isn't just people with endometriosis, but it's people who experience really painful or heavy periods or other menstrual conditions. It's about reimagining the workforce. It needs to come from employers down, developing that comfortable culture to talk about women's health in the workplace, providing support to female staff so they feel comfortable approaching the employer with problems. Being able to have the autonomy and feel empowered to restructure your work around your symptoms."

This restructuring might start with tracking your symptoms each month to see a pattern of when you struggle the most at your job. Do you struggle most with fatigue in the days leading up to your period and/or have a hard time sitting in a chair the first day? These are things to start tracking. When you are able to get a clearer picture of when your symptoms most interfere with your work, you'll be able to present your requests in more specific ways that can help you and your employer come up with a plan. For instance, instead of saying, "I have really bad periods. Can I work from home?," you could say, "This job is really important to me, and I always want to give you my best. I've tracked the days I struggle the most with my endometriosis, and I'd like to work from home or come into work later on those two days each month."

Working from home might not always be an option, especially for physically demanding roles like working on a factory floor, waitressing, or being an ER nurse. But are you able to look at how you might be able to work in more of an administrative role on certain days or change your tasks? It might not always be perfect, but it's worth asking and giving it a shot.

Victoria says it can be a "disclosure dance" of knowing what to share with your employer. She suggests printing off information or studies about how endometriosis affects the workplace. You can share this information with HR or your supervisor before speaking to them, which can take a little pressure off of you if you're already feeling anxious about the conversation. It's been shown that women are less likely to discuss their endo and symptoms if they are concerned that others believe it has emotional origins.[10] Presenting them with the facts and figures can take away some of this worry. On the flip side of this disclosure dance, I asked Sabrina, whom we heard from earlier, if she disclosed her endo to her employer, and she said no. But she shared, "If you don't ask, they're never going to give it to you," and when you do ask, "you don't even have to say why."

Now You.

How has endo impacted your work or career trajectory?

_____

_____

_____

_____

_____

_____

_____

If you are struggling to keep up during certain times of the month, are there ways that you can make changes to your schedule or role at work?

_____

_____

_____

_____

_____

_____

_____

YOUR FIVE-WEEK
ENDO TOOL KIT

Week One: Know Your Endo

Welcome to Week One!

You might be wondering why the first tool is Know Your Endo... *Hello, I picked up this book because I already KNOW or think I have endo. What more do I need to know about it?* But stay with me and don't skip ahead, because Knowing Your Endo is one of the most important tools in your kit. It's the foundational tool from which you'll build your other tools. It's also the tool in which I've seen the most "aha" moments and witnessed the most profound transformations in how people see themselves. And it's an opportunity to create a new level of empathy and compassion for yourself that you didn't think was possible.

In Chapter 2, we defined endometriosis and its symptoms, but this week we're going to dive into how your symptoms make *you* feel. In order to begin to manage your symptoms, you must first learn exactly how they show up in your life. By mastering this new tool, you'll create a new sense of clarity and finally connect the dots between the symptoms and your endo and how you feel on a monthly, weekly, and even daily basis. Connecting those dots can be a game changer both physically *and* mentally.

As an added bonus, learning this tool is bigger than just you. There are so many of us with endo who don't fully understand the extent of how our symptoms impact our lives. If we don't fully understand this impact, how can we expect the people around us to understand it and support us? After truly learning to Know Your Endo and arming yourself with the knowledge and language around it, you'll be able to better advocate for yourself with care providers—and better communicate with your friends and family on how they can support you. It's an extremely powerful tool, and I'm really excited for you to get started.

Actually, wait. Before we get started, there's one more thing I need to tell you. As you work your way through this chapter and complete your worksheets, you may have some big emotions come to the surface. They might even flood the surface. You may have old feelings of sadness you thought you buried, or even a new sense of empowerment that might surprise you. Whether you cry, get pissed off, nervously laugh your way through it, or all of the above . . . that's okay. It's more than okay. Feel it all. It might be uncomfortable at first, but sometimes change can be uncomfortable. Remember that as you begin Week One, there is another friendo out there doing the same exact thing—getting uncomfortable, feeling lots of emotions, and beginning to make change. You're definitely not alone in this process.

What do you wish everyone knew about living with endometriosis?

You can feel fine one day and the next your body can be completely possessed by the illness.

—Diana Falzone

———

In case you skipped it or need a refresher, let's review:

What Is Endometriosis?

Endometriosis in an inflammatory condition in which endometrial-like tissue (similar to the tissue that lines the uterus and is shed during menstruation) is found in other places in the body. It usually involves the ovaries, bowel, or the tissue lining your pelvis, though sometimes it can spread beyond the pelvic region, including but not limited to the appendix, diaphragm, and lungs.

What Are the Symptoms?

Very painful periods (pelvic pain, cramping, lower-back and abdominal pain)*

Pain during ovulation or two weeks after your period

Leg pain or neuralgia (nerve sensations) associated with your cycle

Hip pain and/or back pain

Shoulder/chest pain or shortness of breath with your cycle

Pain during or after sex

Thick blood clots (often dark) with your period

Painful bowel movements or painful urination

Excessive bleeding

Fatigue and chronic pain

Diarrhea and constipation

Bloating

Nausea and vomiting

Urinary frequency, retention, or urgency

Allergies and other immune-related issues

Infertility and pregnancy loss (though many women can still have children)

I wanted to share this list of symptoms again, because the first time I ever saw it, it blew my mind. I had dealt with painful and unexplained

---

* *Not everyone with endometriosis has painful periods. Some people experience periods without pain but experience other symptoms the rest of the month.*

health issues for over two decades—and within seconds of reading the list, all of those issues made sense to me.

Symptom Stories

Let's take urinary frequency and urgency. For as long as I can remember, I could never seem to make it to the bathroom in time. Out of nowhere, a feeling of having TO GO! would hit. When this feeling hit, I'd race to the bathroom doing the "I have to pee" waddle or subtly try to hold my crotch while fast-walking to the bathroom. Nine times out of ten, I'd make it into the bathroom stall. But then I'd struggle with a zipper, button, or hard-to-get-off Spanx, and ultimately pee myself. You have no idea how many pairs of soggy underwear I've thrown away in the bathrooms of stores and restaurants because I wasn't sure what to do with them after peeing myself.

I remember I once went to a fancy party that my husband's work hosted at one of the most well-known and beautiful art museums in the country. And I peed my pants in that well-known and beautiful art museum's bathroom. I was so ashamed wiping the pee up off the floor. After wiping it up, I just stood there with my wet underwear in my hand not knowing what to do. Was it better to walk around with no underwear with the possibility of my skirt flying up and exposing myself *or* talk to my husband's boss wearing pee-soaked underwear? I decided to throw them away in the bathroom and take my chances with the wind. As mortifying as that was, at least I had made it safely to the stall that night. Because there were times when I didn't. I once crouched down in a park pretending to pick flowers while I peed, because there wasn't a bathroom in sight. And there was the time in college when I couldn't find the keys to my dorm fast enough and peed all over the entryway (hoping someone would just chalk it up to a drunk girl in my dorm, before I was able to clean it up).

Sometimes I'd share my pee stories with my family and friends.

Because, in a weird way, it made me feel better to laugh it off and try to normalize it in some way. By sharing, I wanted to reframe these stories as one of my weird quirks or another funny thing I did and not that I was a gross person. But, even when they'd laugh, I could tell they didn't think it was totally normal to pee in the middle of a park while pretending to pick flowers. I also got a lot of advice: maybe I waited too long to go pee or needed to go before I left the house (like a toddler who is potty training). A doctor once told me I needed to drink more water throughout the day. But none of them (nor I) knew that urinary urgency was a symptom of my endometriosis. When I was finally diagnosed and saw that this was a symptom on the list, it changed how I saw myself. I wasn't a gross person—and it had nothing to do with poor planning skills.

Let's look at another person's symptom story. Before she was diagnosed, Taylor was a very sporadic planner because of her fatigue. She could only make plans when she wasn't tired, but it felt like she was tired all the time. Her friends thought of her as being all-or-nothing when it came to hanging out. She was either totally in or totally out—which made her feel really misunderstood. It wasn't that she didn't want to be with her family and friends, it's that she was just too exhausted.

What is your endo motto?

What doesn't kill me better run!

—Meg Allan Cole

Taylor's story isn't uncommon. So many of us with endo are sporadic planners, serial cancelers, or we simply give up on planning in the first place. When we do this, it makes us feel like we're letting down the people around us. When Taylor was finally diagnosed with endometriosis at the age of thirty-four, it all began to make sense. She had so much fatigue because of her endometriosis. And she felt much more understood.

Because of these stories and the countless others I've heard over the years, sharing endometriosis symptoms is something I'm really passionate about. I've shared this list of symptoms hundreds of times—during talks I've given, in interviews, with friends and family, and even with strangers at parties. Knowing these symptoms is a huge component of raising awareness and getting people diagnosed sooner. But it's also a way for us to get to know ourselves better. It's one thing to see a symptom on a list and think, *I have that!* But it's another to take the time to bring that symptom to life and truly articulate how it feels in *your* body, how it has impacted your life, and how it makes you feel about yourself.

It's time to grab a pen again and write down your symptom stories. Don't be shy or hold back as you write. I just told you that I peed on the floor at a fancy museum, so anything goes. No one else has to see these answers unless you want them to.

When you begin to work through this list, it's important to remember that you may experience one or all of these symptoms. But this is not an endo competition, and there are no prizes for who has it the worst. It really doesn't matter how many symptoms you suffer from. One symptom (no matter how severe) is all it takes for you to feel discomfort or affect your self-worth. It's also important to remember that this is not about creating a list to show what a "mess" you are and using it as permission to give up. No matter how bad you might feel right now, you are not a lost cause. In the weeks ahead, we'll be working together to help manage some of these symptoms (and maybe say goodbye to some forever).

Now You.

Check off any symptoms you have experienced:

☐ Very painful periods (pelvic pain, cramping, lower-back and abdominal pain)

☐ Leg, hip, or back pain

☐ Pain during or after sex

☐ Thick blood clots (often dark) with your period

☐ Painful bowel movements or painful urination

☐ Urinary frequency, retention, or urgency

☐ Excessive bleeding

☐ Fatigue and chronic pain

☐ Diarrhea and constipation

☐ Bloating

☐ Nausea and vomiting

☐ Infertility

Are there any additional symptoms you experience that aren't on this list?

Go through each checked-off symptom, think about your symptom stories, and answer the following questions (grab an extra piece of paper or a journal if you need more space).

How have these symptoms impacted your life and/or shaped how you feel about yourself?

_____

_____

_____

_____

_____

Do you feel in control of these symptoms?

_____

_____

_____

_____

_____

_____

Have you tried to manage them in the past?

_____

_____

_____

_____

_____

Looking at your answers, how you do feel? Sad? Mad? More compassion for yourself? Fired up to make change?

_____

_____

_____

_____

_____

Like I said, it's normal to feel some big emotions right now. Doing the work you just did was a lot to take in!

Your mission this week is to sit with these emotions, come back to these pages, and fill in more whenever you need to. Take some time to let everything marinate and sink in. For the remainder of the week, use the additional box below to note any symptoms you experience, any feelings or emotions that come up with them, and how they impact your day-to-day life.

I'll see you back here next week.

_____

_____

_____

_____

Week Two: Stress Management

Before We Begin

Before we start talking about how to manage stress, I think it's important to define the stress we're talking about here. Because there's definitely good stress and bad stress. Big stress and little stress. There are so many different types of stressors in our lives that it can be incredibly difficult to define. My favorite definition comes from research psychologist Kelly McGonigal's book *The Upside of Stress.* She defines stress as "what arises when something you care about is at stake."[1] I love that line, "something you care about." Because during stressful times, we can get so caught up in the mental and physical reactions and the escalation of our stress that we lose sight of the very thing we care about in the first place—the thing that we care about that is at stake. Kelly's definition enables us to take a step back and give more compassion toward our stress. But as many of us have experienced, that's easier said than done.

While stress isn't a symptom of endo, they seem to go hand in hand. It feels like a chicken-and-egg situation *or* a catch-22 *or* some other popular adage I can't think of right now. Are we more stressed because of our endo *or* do our endo symptoms create more stress? The answer is that both are true. For most of us, stress and endo are a package deal. So much so, it might feel hard to separate the two.

We commonly get stressed over money: "I'm so stressed about my credit card bill right now!" and over work and school: "This project is turning me into a ball of stress!" and our relationships: "My mom's texts are stressing me out right now!" But it's rare that we talk about how our endo is stressing us out. I've never once said, "This cyst is really stressing me out today!" or "Damn, this fatigue has got me stressed!" Why? For starters, we've been conditioned not to talk about it. Most people in our lives are cool with us complaining about the common stressors of work, money, and relationships. But our endo and periods? Not as much. We've learned through people's facial expressions, body language, and dramatic interruptions ("La la la! Gross! Stop talking about that!") that they're not interested in hearing what we have to say. So we stop sharing, and we repress our stress and never give it a voice. And unlike your endometriosis, those other common stressors usually come with an opportunity to alleviate them.

With work, you could talk to HR about the issues you're having or even look for a new job. With money, you can try to find ways to spend less and save more. And with your relationships, there are ways to work on communicating better with whomever's texts are stressing you out. You do have some sense of agency and control over these things. But with endo, no matter how hard you try, it's always there. You can't switch bodies like you can switch your job—or block your endo's number, like you can with those stress-texters. Having endo is out of your control. And that lack of control only strengthens the marriage between endo and stress, a.k.a. Strendo (the stress and endo dynamic duo).

In an article from the *Journal of Molecular Medicine*, Dr. Bettina Toth summarized the findings: "The wealth of published evidence supporting that (1) endometriosis is associated with a poor quality of life and high stress perception; (2) endometriosis is an inflammatory disease, and (3) stress and poor quality of life may cause inflammation, strongly suggested that women with endometriosis are stuck between a rock and a hard place within the vicious circle of high stress perception, inflammation, and disease progression."[2]

That "vicious cycle" is what we need to stop. In order to do that, we first need to acknowledge our stress and give it a voice. We can then begin to separate the bond between our endo and stress and our stress from our endo. By doing this, we can start to reframe it—and also target our stress with practical management practices. During this week, you will discover ways to start to have more compassion for yourself, manage your stress better, and begin the divorce process for one of the most problematic couples of all time (goodbye, Strendo).

Giving Your Stress a Voice

Growing up, many people have cute nicknames that their friends and family give them. Maybe a nod to a cuddly animal they resemble or a loving term of endearment. Well, my nickname was Stressica. I was always stressed about everything. Name something and I could find a way to worry and obsess over it. And not in a low-key way. My stress was debilitating and paralyzing. It affected everything I did, and I couldn't seem to get a handle on it.

I stressed about being stressed. I stressed about not being stressed enough. I thought this was just the way I was built, that I would forever be Stressica. But as I began to become more mindful about how my stress made me feel, I surprised myself—and the stressed-out me began to change. The more I started to take an active role in creating lifestyle tools for myself—the way I ate, the way I thought, and the time I devoted to finding calm for my body . . . the less stress and worry I felt.

Now, I'm not saying I'm all zen all the time. I still get little stress bursts about money and work deadlines. And the last five years of my life have been unusually chaotic and, at times, traumatic. I became a mom, moved states, survived two hurricanes (and a flood), had two major surgeries, wrote a book, my grandmother and both of my pets passed away, and my stepmother had two near-death experiences (she survived being run over by a bus *and* necrotizing fasciitis in a span of four months). Needless to say, it was a wild five years of many ups and downs. The old Stressica would have completely lost it and become paralyzed in the stress and fear, but the not-so-Stressica, armed with her new tools, managed to get through it all, with some sanity intact.

Was I able to get through it completely unscathed? Of course not. There were moments that were awful. I could only do my best, and there were times that it just wasn't possible to stop for a mindful stroll around the block. I remember, during the chaos of evacuating for hurricane number one, we prepped our house to leave; packed enough food, socks, and underwear for the undetermined time we were going to be away; wrangled a toddler and two cats into a car; and drove for hours to get out of the hurricane's way.

During this time, I did my best to remain calm, didn't cry, and pushed through it all. As much as I was doing a good job at not visibly freaking out, I was also doing a really good job at catastrophizing about all the chaos in my head. *Would my neighbors, who weren't able to leave, be okay? Would our house get destroyed in the hurricane? How much would our insurance help us with the damage? Wait, did we have insurance for this?! Where would we live as we rebuild our house? Wait. Seriously. Did we have insurance to even cover a rebuild?* I had visions of my husband and me standing in a pile of rubble, searching for any photos we could salvage. I was glued to the news, and all the images of destroyed homes in the neighboring cities only made my thoughts worse. A couple of days after we evacuated (and a couple of days catastrophizing), my period started and I suffered some of the worst cramps I'd had in years. My endo let me know it wasn't happy about all that stress, and I was creating more pain for myself.

As we learned earlier in this book, catastrophizing can lead to increased pain. Heba Shaheed, a physical therapist living in Australia who specializes in working with people who have endometriosis (and has endo herself), explains that when we are stressed and/or thinking negative thoughts, we are sending fear-driven messages into our brains. Our limbic system (the part of our brain that controls fear, memories, and our emotional and physical responses) goes into over-drive, which can then send more messages to our brain that we're in danger. By doing this, it can actually create more pain and exacerbate our symptoms.

I was definitely creating more pain for my-self. My endo let me know it wasn't happy about all that stress—and it hurt like hell. But as much as it hurt, I remember lying in bed and feeling weirdly proud of myself. Feeling that pain reminded me how far I had come since my Stressica days, when this pain was a monthly occurrence. Those cramps were a

Which words or phrases do you most overuse about your endo?

I'm fine.

—*April Christina*

beast, but I was able to lie there knowing it was temporary. While I couldn't control Mother Nature, I could control how I helped my body through it all. I was also reminded of just how important my stress-management tools were to my mental and physical health (they worked!). As soon as this pain faded, I would start practicing my stress-management tools again, and I knew I would feel better the next time my period came around. And that felt empowering.

That stressful and traumatic five-year span included very extreme circumstances. But just because you aren't driving away from a hurri-cane or had a loved one pass away doesn't mean that your stress is triv-ial. It's important not to "grade our stress," as Dr. Elizabeth Stanley discusses in her book *Widen the Window: Training Your Brain and Body to Thrive during Stress and Recover from Trauma*. Dr. Stanley explains that our brains have developed ways of judging our stress and trauma compared to other people. After comparing, we tend to deem our own stress of being worthy or not.[3]

This is something I found myself doing during the most difficult times in the past five years. I'd ask myself, *Should I be this upset when so many other people have it far worse than me?* The reality is, your stress is *your* stress. It doesn't matter how it compares to other people's.

So now, I want to ask you: What are the biggest stressors in your life? What are the things you care about most that are at stake, and why do you care about them? Remember to try not to compare them to anybody else's stress. Whatever you are feeling is valid. Really sit down and think about your stressors, and if you are able to, identify how that stress presents itself in your body and how your body reacts. For example, do you feel uneasy or does your heart race when you're around certain judgmental family members or friends? Do your period cramps go off the charts during stressful life events? Big or small, please list all the things that have consistently or recently made you feel stressed and why you care about them. Do your best to remember how they made your body feel. It's okay if you aren't yet sure about how you react to stress. You can come back to this page anytime you want to record it, once you begin to recognize it. The key is to start giving your stress a voice so you can begin to manage it better.

Now You.

Record your stressors and how they make you feel.

_____

_____

_____

_____

_____

_____

Entering the Cycle

When I spoke about the vicious cycle of stress, endo, and inflammation with integrative physician and women's health expert Dr. Aviva Romm, she explained that it's not about figuring out where to *break* the vicious cycle (it was important to her to not use "breaking" as the defining language here). It's about deciding where to *enter* into the cycle and start to heal and soothe the immune, endocrine, and stress-response systems so that they will all calm down together.

It's not just about calming down your immune system, either. Dr. Romm explains that there's cognitive stress involved in being diagnosed with endometriosis.

I'm not sure about you, but the moment I got home from the hospital after my diagnosis, I went online to see what this meant for my future, and I quickly entered the dark vortex of endo gloom and doom. *There's no cure! You can't have children! Sex hurts! You will probably need a hysterectomy!* I was supposed to be relieved that I had gotten a diagnosis, but in some ways, I wished I hadn't gotten one. It made me feel hopeless, and I had a hard time finding anyone who would tell me, *"It's gonna be okay."*

There's an underlying stress from the uncertainty of when your symptoms will decide to present themselves, not to mention the many unknowns you are likely to face: whether you can have children or not; if you'll need (another) surgery; if a cyst will come back and rupture again; if your pain and symptoms will make an appearance during your important presentation at work, the vacation you've planned for a year, or your sister's wedding. All of that worrying would give most people anxiety (with or without endo). And then tack on the stress of having to tell your boss you can't make the presentation, having to cancel the vacation you dreamed about, or letting your sister down on her big day . . . and there's a whole other level of stress. These unknowns can also feel like a vicious cycle.

So how do we enter this vicious cycle and begin to repair it? We can't truly learn to manage our stress until we're able to learn and begin to practice self-compassion.

What Does Self-Compassion Mean?

When I first stumbled upon self-compassion work, I thought, *Here we go again . . . yet another new practice that's going to tell me that all my problems will be solved if I stand in front of a mirror and tell myself how pretty and smart I am. Not for me.* I had tried doing positive-affirmation work before, and it just never clicked. Maybe I didn't do it long enough, or maybe the fact that I found it a little cheesy limited its potential for me. I'm not really sure—I just know I didn't like how it made me feel.

But as I started learning more about self-compassion, I realized just how wrong I was about it. Self-compassion isn't becoming my own personal hype man to increase my self-esteem. That's not what it's about at all. By definition, self-compassion is applying to myself the level of kindness I extend to others. It is creating more awareness about what I need in moments of stress and pain and giving those things to myself. And beyond that, it's about giving that to myself without judgment.

If you're thinking that the idea of self-compassion isn't necessarily a new one, you're right—it's been around for thousands of years. Compassion is a key theme of Buddhism, and there are hundreds of thousands of compassion-inspired quotes from Mother Teresa to Sharon Salzberg to the Buddha himself. So, what's so different here? Until pretty recently, we've historically looked at compassion through a spirituality and hippie-dippie-self-help lens. But in the last decade, research (pioneered by the work of Dr. Kristin Neff) has begun to scientifically measure the profound impact of self-compassion on our bodies, brains, and overall well-being.

Sabrina Vogler, a self-compassion teacher trained by Dr. Neff, explains that our nervous system is designed to eavesdrop on everything that's going on in our brains and the way that we take in the world.

When Sabrina shared this with me, I thought it was a little sad (and creepy) to think that my nervous system was eavesdropping on all the self-loathing and judgmental thinking I had been doing all these years. But Sabrina explains that it's not our fault that we're constantly judging, because it's our brain's default reaction. "Our default mode has kept us alive. If you were being chased by a predator and you were in this state of, *Well I'm open-minded about this, and maybe the saber-toothed tiger isn't very hungry today. All is probably going to be okay,* in that moment you're not going to survive. The fact that we default to judging has kept us alive because we judge good or bad, safe or danger."

Where the problem lies is if every time that we become over-whelmed (and I'm not talking being chased by a tiger—I'm talking about the overwhelm we feel about our bodies and pain), that intense judgment can become our fixed state. This fixed state can be incredibly problematic for people with a chronic condition. "Anytime you have the word 'chronic,' there's also going to be some conditioning that happens in the brain around the nature of being chronic," Sabrina explains. But there is hope for us. Sabrina says that our brains are "incredibly adaptive," and when "we shift our relationship with our default state, then our relationship with stress changes." By using self-compassion, we have the power to change our default state and what our nervous system is listening to. Pretty amazing, right?

So how do we begin to use self-compassion and shift our default state? In *Self-Compassion: The Proven Power of Being Kind to Yourself,* Dr. Neff shares that the first step is to stop and recognize our suffering. She explains, "We can't be moved by our pain if we don't acknowledge that it exists in the first place."[4] This is easier said than done, of course. Because sometimes we don't feel like we have the luxury to stop and recognize what we're going through, let alone give ourselves the care that we need.

People with endo are the queens/kings of pushing through. Cramps? Push through. Depression? Push through. Period just soaked through your underwear? Roll up a wad of toilet paper, stuff it in there, and push through. Most of us push through because we have to. If you call off work, you might lose your job. If you miss a test at school, you might fail that course. If you don't get out of bed, your child will not eat. The truth is that you can love the idea of acknowledging pain and asking for what you need all day long. The issue is having the time and mental freedom to provide yourself with this very well-deserved luxury.

Using Self-Compassion

So, how can we start using self-compassion if we feel that we have obstacles that get in the way of it? Sabrina explains: "Self-compassion asks, at any given moment, *'What am I experiencing? And what do I need?'* Introducing those two questions in the form of a new habit is a way of activating your own internal caregiver. You are explicitly messaging your nervous system and telling your physical body that there is now an internal caregiver who is aware and supportive. And your nervous system will receive that messaging." She went on to illustrate this with an example. "Let's say you get out of bed, and you notice that your body is hurting. Self-compassion might cause you to get out of bed in a different way and say, 'I'm feeling cold, so why don't I put something warm on my body.' This will send the message to yourself (and your nervous system) that support is here. The quality of talking to yourself while you're going through those steps and saying, 'You know what, dearest? This does feel like a very tough moment and I see it clearly. Because there's not a lot of extra time right now. How can we make the most of this opportunity to offer you support?'"

Since I've begun practicing self-compassion, it's truly changed how I approach my endo. I actually remember the very first moment I ever practiced it. I woke up on the first day of my period feeling really bloated and achy. I was on solo-parent duty because my husband was out of town, and I had a packed day of back-to-back meetings and interviews. I had to be *on*, and there were zero opportunities to let my body rest that day. Before self-compassion, I would have judged and questioned if I had done something wrong to contribute to my bloat and pain. I would have been embarrassed to show up to my meetings with my fatigue face (not technically a medical condition, but I'm pretty sure you know that tired face I'm talking about). I would have pushed through it all with so much force that I'd have been wiped out by the end of the night.

But with self-compassion, I remember waking up and thinking, *Okay, you're bloated today because of your endo, and I know that really sucks. You also don't feel like you look your best and that stinks, too. But I want to care for you. What can we do to make it better?* At that moment, I took a deep breath, and found my loosest pair of underwear, which put less pressure on my bloated belly. While my son ate breakfast, I lay on the ground next to him and raised my legs against the wall to stretch and give my body a tiny rest. For my meetings, I wore my flowiest dress and these over-the-top colorful shoes (I didn't feel pretty that day, but those colorful shoes were). They were small acts of care, but they were big signals to my nervous system that the negative and catastrophizing signals it had been receiving all those years were beginning to change. Moving forward, I would be applying to myself the level of kindness I extend to others.

I'm not saying this work is easy in the beginning. It takes practice. Sabrina explains that, at first, it's normal to feel like you're putting your left shoe on your right foot. But we can change. We can be kinder to ourselves with practice. And you know the coolest part? Sabrina says, "The compassion centers of the brain—and we have a lot of neuroscience to back this up—are literally inexhaustible. So, for all that is unsustainable about living with chronic illness, compassion is inexhaustible. You are literally tapping into a well that will never run dry."

We're just skimming the surface on self-compassion here. If you want to learn more about it, check out Dr. Neff's book and website on self-compassion for free guided meditations and exercises, and do a search for self-compassion teachers, like Sabrina, near you.

Stress-Management Tools

Okay! We have identified stressors and deemed them worthy, we understand that we need to end the vicious cycle, and we understand how self-compassion can actually change how we process pain. Now we're ready for some practical stress-management tools. While you're not going to have to practice these all at one time, please make sure to read through each one—even if you don't think you'd be into it. They might inspire you to think of an entirely new tool, or you may surprise yourself and see that you do want to give it a try.

Mindfulness

In addition to self-compassion, I believe mindfulness is the second backbone to creating successful stress-management practices. Not only have researchers found that consistent mindfulness practices have been shown to change the gray matter in our brains, but the effects can be felt well beyond the moments we practice them—and help with stress, depression, and anxiety.[5] You might be thinking that this is all leading up to me telling you that you must meditate. It's not. If you love meditation or have been curious about starting it, go for it! Mindfulness and breath-based meditation practices have significantly changed people's lives, and that's incredible. But not everyone is ready for or capable of meditation right now. It might be something you need to build up to, or you may decide that other mindfulness practices are more your style.

Dr. Elizabeth Stanley explains that many assume that when we practice breath-based meditation, the sensations with breathing will be neutral. But for those of us who have traumatic histories of prolonged, chronic stress, when we bring our attention to the sensations of breathing, there is the possibility of tapping into this unresolved chronic stress and trauma. She says this is why many people experience restlessness, anxiety, panic attacks, shallow breathing, nausea, and other sensations while doing breath-based meditation.

For many of us, endo has been a chronic stressor in our lives and may have caused significant trauma by way of miscarriage, surgery, ER visits, or pain so bad you black out, among other physical and emotional traumas. This, of course, can be compounded by other trauma you may have experienced that is not connected to your endometriosis, such as a sexual assault, the death of a family member, or exposure to violence, among other painful events. The heartbreaking thing is that we're so used to stress and trauma from our endo (or we've been made to believe that it's all in our heads), we don't often recognize what we've gone through or are currently going through. Melissa, the friendo living in Canada whom we heard from earlier, says she was reluctant to speak to me for this book because she wasn't sure she really had anything to contribute or share. That is, until her best friend reminded Melissa that her pain had been invalidated for years until a visit to the ER revealed that she had a cyst the size of a grapefruit. Hearing Melissa say this brought tears to my eyes. Of course she had experienced trauma, and of course she had a story to share.

Finding Your Version of Mindfulness

If you're not ready for meditation or have felt those sensations of anxiety, restlessness, and panic attacks while trying to practice it, that's okay. There's absolutely nothing wrong with you, and you can still create more mindfulness in your life. Dr. Stanley says, "Mindfulness is a quality of the way our minds work," and it doesn't have to be practiced solely through meditation. "When we're learning to regulate ourselves and when we're learning to cultivate mindfulness, we need to do it mindfully. We need to do it with awareness of our body's current limits. That's why picking intentional targets that are going to be neutral for us, even if we're sitting on a bunch of unresolved chronic stress and trauma, that's a really skillful choice." It can start with paying attention to sights and sounds around us: "Washing dishes, feeling the suds and warm water under your hands. Brushing your teeth and feeling all of those bristles—all the little movements bristled against your teeth and against your gums and the taste of the toothpaste." It's truly about starting to become more fully present during certain moments of your day.

Mindful walking is another way to start practicing mindfulness. Dr. Stanley shares, "My favorite mindfulness practice when someone does not feel ready to sit down to meditate is walking mindfully in nature. Because nature is so regulating, it can help us regulate." At the end of this chapter, I will share Dr. Stanley's guide for mindful walking and how we're going to put it into practice this week.

Last, grounding yourself is another helpful mindfulness tool. Grounding is the practice of focusing on the present moment and tapping into your physical body and/or surroundings. Which might sound complicated, but it can simply be taking time to focus on the feeling of your butt in a chair or holding an object and directing your attention to how its textures feel in your hand. Dr. Stanley says grounding works because "it's a way to help cue the survival brain to appraise the situation as safe." By doing this, we can help turn our stress arousal off.

Give it a try the next time you're in bed with racing thoughts about the day ahead or catastrophizing your pain. Start by lying there and decide that for thirty seconds, you will focus on the weight of your body. Focus on how your body feels against the mattress, the heels of your feet at the bottom of the bed, and your head pressing into the pillow. That thirty seconds might turn into a minute or maybe three. Ground yourself until you can feel your body and mind start to calm down. It's a simple practice, but it can be extremely powerful.

Again, if you are a master meditator already, keep it up!

If you have struggled with it in the past, mindful walking and grounding are a great place to start. Kundalini chanting and Ziva meditation are also worth checking out if you have had issues with breath-based meditation. They can be a nice entry into more traditional meditation practices.

Stress-Management Hobbies

When you start to think about creating stress-management hobbies, it's a good time to revisit the things you loved to do as a kid—the time when your younger self was creative without fear of judgment of what you were creating and put all your focus into what was right in front of you. That type of focus, for your grown-up self, can be a way to distract you from your pain.

One of my favorite stress-busting tools are jigsaw puzzles. There is something about them that always chills me out and calms my mind. Amanda Kahle, co-founder of the puzzle company Inner Piece, says puzzles are an incredible stress-management tool because "we live in a world that embraces multitasking, when really our brains are much healthier when we take time to focus on one thing at a time. Working on a jigsaw puzzle uses both the logic and creative sides of your brain, simultaneously. Focusing on a single task like this for at least fifteen minutes has shown to have meditative-like benefits, which releases stress and anxiety, as well as improving brain health and performance over time." It becomes more difficult to focus on your stress when you're focused on the task in front of you.

In addition to puzzles, papier-mâché, knitting, crocheting, painting, doodling, coloring, sculpting, and playing an instrument can have the same effect. One friendo told me she crochets whenever she's feeling stressed. She said she loves that it keeps her hands busy, which helps her stay off her phone, too (something else that gives her stress).

If you're wondering how you could possibly find more time in your day to sit down and leisurely do a puzzle or color, I get it. But you know that time you spend scrolling on your phone when you wake up in the morning? Mosey on over to a puzzle or creative hobby and spend those minutes there instead. Same thing goes for the minutes you spend in bed at night messing around on your phone or watching TV. Getting creative and having mindful hobbies can be meditative *and* counts as a form of solitude (which you're about to read about next), a real BOGO stress-management tool.

Unplug + Reconnect

The majority of us are constantly connected to media—and I'm not just talking about the social kind. It's texts, emails, podcasts, audiobooks, streaming movies and shows on our phones, regular old movies and shows on TV, video games, online news and celebrity gossip sites, and I'm sure I'm forgetting something. Yes, a lot of these things can bring us joy, help us relax after a long day, and no doubt help us feel more connected. But the problem is that we're constantly consuming information and not giving our brains a break. Cal Newport, computer science professor and author of *Digital Minimalism: Choosing a Focused Life in a Noisy World*, calls our constant connectivity "solitude deprivation,"[6] which he defines as "a state in which you spend close to zero time alone with your own thoughts and free from input from other minds." This state of constant connectivity with no alone time can cause anxiety and depression and can actually make us feel less connected.

It's important to define what Cal means by solitude, because he says it isn't necessarily physical separation from others. For example, heading to a remote cabin in the woods for a week alone but still checking social media the whole time you're there is not solitude. But being on a crowded subway or plane without checking your phone or listening to music or a podcast is.

The scary part about solitude is that a lot of us don't want to be alone with our thoughts, and that's why we're seeking out the distractions in the first place. How many times have you noticed that when you're waiting in your car in traffic, early for an appointment, or have another opportunity to be alone with your thoughts, you reach for your phone as soon as a thought emerges that you don't want to deal with? We're also constantly seeking out ways to never feel "bored." The other day I overheard a man at the grocery store telling his friend that now that he has a waterproof phone, he'd been catching up on his favorite shows in the shower. In the shower. One of the last (I thought) guaranteed spaces for some healthy boredom and solitude.

Cal says that you can find more solitude simply by taking walks without your phone. No podcasts? No music? No talking with your best friend to pass the time? No. Just you and your thoughts. This is the second vote for mindful walking in this chapter! As I said, I'll be sharing how to do this soon.

I understand that finding solitude can be hard with family, school, a demanding job, and/or not wanting to be alone with your thoughts. So maybe it's starting with sitting alone in the bathroom for fifteen minutes (lock the door, if you need to), or cooking without listening to music or podcasts, or simply sitting in a waiting room or in traffic without pulling out your phone. Heba Shaheed suggests that after driving home at the end of the day, stop in front of your house and sit in your car for five minutes and just focus on letting any tension in your body go. I love this, because if you do this every day, you're getting at least thirty minutes of solitude each week. Solitude might feel uncomfortable at first, but it can be a critical piece of the puzzle to calming your body and mind.

Find Your People

"The sense of being alone in our suffering is one of the biggest barriers to transforming stress" (more words of wisdom from Kelly McGongial's *Upside of Stress*).[7] I thought about this line so much after reading it, because having endo can be an incredibly isolating and lonely place to live. You can have the most supportive partner or family in the world but still feel alone in your disease. *How could they possibly understand what I'm going through? How dare they give me health advice when they've never had a bad period in their life!* Those feelings of isolation can lead to depression and poor health and can affect your physical activity.[8] But I don't think the solution is to shut these people out. I believe the solution is to welcome new people in. It can be a game changer to find *your people* (or even a single person)—ones who can support or understand what you're going through.

Of course, the easiest way of doing this is to hop online and find endo social media groups and forums. I've heard from so many friendos who benefit from being able to share in those spaces. A lot of them are shy or feel uncomfortable sharing, while online feels like a safe space for them to be open about what they are going through. But this isn't for everyone.

As important as it is to find your people, it's just as important to figure out the way that you like to connect with them. Personally, I don't love big social media groups. The empath in me feels a lot of sadness hearing everyone's stories and the pain that sometimes comes with them. Also, there's no guarantee that people will know how to respond to your story or even see what you're sharing at all. After one of my Know Your Endo online course sessions, one member told me, "I was desperately seeking women I could have some sort of community with, and especially to talk about endo infertility. I actually didn't even complete the class because no one acknowledged any of my comments in the community group page, and it left me feeling worse." When she shared this with me over a year after the course was over, it broke my heart. With the influx of messages and sharing during the course, I'd completely missed her posts. If I had seen them, I would have given her the care and compassion she needed. She ended up feeling more alone, which is the opposite of how I wanted the group to make her feel.

If groups aren't your thing, that doesn't mean you can't find your people. A lot of cities have meetup groups and events for people with endo (with real-life humans in a room together!). There are endo marches and conferences every year that you can volunteer for, and meet others by attending. You can also use those online social groups to your advantage. Put the word out that you are looking for people in your city (or surrounding cities) with endo. Plan a potluck together, go out for dinner, or meet up for coffee. If you can't find anyone close by, find the person with whom you connect best in your group and ask if they want to start doing monthly video chats or calls, or simply start texting funny cat memes to each other.

What have you gained because of your endo?

A built-in support group. And also a strong desire to rip out my uterus at least once a month.

—Ashlae W.

Last, finding your people doesn't mean that those people have to have endometriosis. Endo might be the last thing that you want to talk or think about, but it's still important to find meaningful connections to feel less alone. A great way to do that is by seeking out people who have the same passions or hobbies as you do (or ones you want to try). Whether it's reading, knitting, DIY projects, bowling, gardening, cooking, video games, writing, spirituality, hiking, and so on, there is most likely a group for it (online and off). Sometimes it can feel really freeing and therapeutic to create, play, and learn with other like-minded people who don't know your health issues or backstory. You can be whoever you want to be in that time together.

I understand that all of this is easier said than done. There are times when your fatigue or cramps might get the best of you, and there's no chance you'll be able to meet up with your new book club or endo walking group. It won't always be perfect, but we must do our best to find our people (or person) to battle the burden of loneliness and isolation that comes with living with a chronic condition. And if that burden ever becomes too much, it's important to seek help.

Movement

The act of stretching, walking, biking, bouncing, or foam rolling can help reduce stress in significant ways. We'll be talking about how movement plays a role in stress management in Chapter 7, but there was no way I couldn't mention it here, too. This week we'll be practicing mindful walking, so you can get a head start on moving your body before we dive deep into the topic in the pages ahead.

Sleep

We've all heard how important it is to sleep. It can help manage stress, regulate our mood, and make us more productive. We can read all day long about why sleep is good, but that doesn't solve the problem of how to get more. This is also a tricky one, because if you're battling fatigue, no amount of sleep ever feels like enough. A lot of us work late and wake up early, have human alarm clocks (kids) that go off whenever they choose, or battle insomnia. Sometimes we can only do our best, but it's also important to take stock of your sleep habits and surroundings to see if there is something you can tweak to make better.

Three questions to ask yourself:

What Are You Doing Once You Get in Bed?

I think most of us have been guilty of staying up too late because we're in bed lurking on social media, online window-shopping, or watching "just one more episode." I'm not going to tell you to not do these things—watching a favorite show in bed after a long workday can feel like the greatest reward ever. But we do need to be mindful of when (and how often) we practice these behaviors. If you know you want to spend some time watching TV before bed, start your bedtime routine a little earlier and limit how many shows you watch. You can turn off the autoplay function on most streaming services (so it doesn't automatically play the next episode and you make that decision for yourself). Make a rule that you can't look at social media in bed. You know the reasons why you're staying up late better than anyone. Try setting up some new boundaries based on your habits and be more mindful of them.

If You Have Children, Can You Work Out Ways to Find More Sleep?
You might be the designated parent on breakfast duty every morning (even on the weekends) or you're the one who gets up in the middle of the night to feed/change/figure out why someone is crying. As you're probably very aware, these two things can really impact your sleep. If possible, have a conversation with your partner about sharing this responsibility. Ask to alternate days of who wakes up in the morning or at night. If this is not possible, see if they can take over on the first few days of your period (when your body can use all the sleep it can get). For single parents or people who work night shifts, this can be a lot harder. But can you seek out trusted family members or friends who can watch your kid(s) one night a month? Could you do a slumber party swap with another single parent you know who could use some extra sleep, too? Every parent has a different budget and circumstances when it comes to childcare, so just do your best to ask for help and get creative to find more sleep for yourself.

Is Your Bedroom/Home Set Up for Good Sleep?
Your sleep environment can also impact your sleep. Certain triggers can keep us up—from how messy your bedroom is to the brightness of the room. It's helpful to identify the triggers that aren't helping your sleep and find solutions to fix them. If your room is super bright, try an eye mask. If there's a lot of noise outside your window at night or your neighbors keep you up, use a white noise app or buy a sound machine. I used to lie paralyzed in bed at night with the fear of someone breaking in. And any sound in my house would send me into a spiral of anxiety and lead to some pretty intense bouts of insomnia. I'd get so scared some nights, I'd put chairs in front of my bedroom door to block any

potential intruders, which is pretty much the most ineffective DIY alarm system ever. After decades of this fear, I finally invested in a real alarm system for my home, and it's the best investment I've ever made for my sleep. Scan your bedroom and see how you might be able to upgrade it for better sleep—whether that's simply picking your clothes up off the floor or getting an eye mask to help block out light.

A final note on sleep: do your best to not stress about your sleep and all the "right" ways to do it. Stressing about your sleep can only lead to less sleep, which can lead to more stress. And on and on. Be honest with yourself about your nighttime habits and see if there is any room for improvement, and always remember to follow the endo sleep motto: get as much as you can, when you can, however you can.

Watch + Read Nice Things

It's really hard to turn on the television or go online and not see violence or sadness, both real or fictionalized. Constantly feeding your brain these images can impact your stress levels and sleep, especially if you're a more sensitive or empathic person. You might not even realize how much it's impacting you until you cut it out. Try to consume positive stories and what I like to call "nice shows." Nice shows do not include murder, violence, and/or terrifying clowns who are designed to keep you up at night. I often get teased about my nice-show choices because they seem cheesy and are nothing but fluff. But I don't care. I enjoy ending a show or movie with a smile and feeling less stressed, and I swear my endo is happier because of it.

Therapy

Living with endometriosis can come with a lot of complicated emotions, and working with a trained therapist can be incredibly healing. For some it could be working through the shame you feel around sex, anxiety about infertility, or just having someone to talk to about your "why me?"

moments. I cannot stress enough the importance of talking to someone outside of your friends and family, someone who is trained to help you.

I understand that not all of us have the means to do this. If cost is an issue, call your insurance company and see how much they cover for mental-health visits, and choose a therapist in your network. If you don't have insurance, some therapists will work on a sliding scale, and there are some online therapy services that offer free sessions. Working with a therapist can give you a better framework for coping with your physical and emotional pain and can be a consistent and reliable source of help in your life (something that many of us struggle to find).

Ready?

I can think of a dozen more ways to manage stress, but these are a good place to start. And it's time to put them into practice!

Your mission this week is to use more self-compassion, find your entry point into the Strendo cycle, follow this week's stress-management guide, and believe that *you can* start to calm your system down by managing your stress. Yes, having endo is out of control. Yes, we can't always control all the stress that comes our way. But we *can* empower ourselves to control how we deal with it.

How to Do Mindful Walking

Before Dr. Stanley gave me the instructions for this mindful-walking practice, she wanted to note that "this is not mindful walking the way it's taught at monasteries or on retreats where you're walking super slow but walking at a regular pace outside and just enjoying and sensing the nature around you." This also doesn't mean that you have to go walk in a forest preserve or a fancy butterfly sanctuary. You can do this walk around your block, city, neighborhood, a local park, or anyplace you can find a bit of nature.

Step One: Leave your phone at home, if you can. If you can't, put it in your pocket or bag and turn off any distracting notifications. There will be no podcasts, music, or catch-ups with friends on this walk.

Step Two: Go outside.

Step Three: You're going to walk and focus on different target objects. Walk at a regular pace for thirty seconds and pay attention to the things you're seeing around you. Maybe it's a giant tree or a rogue weed emerging from the cracks of the sidewalk. Next, for about thirty seconds, pay attention to what you're hearing around you—maybe it's the sound of birds chirping or a jackhammer in the distance. For the next thirty seconds, pay attention to the movement of your arms, the motion of them swinging while you walk. Finally, for another thirty seconds, pay attention to the way your feet touch the ground with each step. Rotate your focus every thirty seconds from the sights, sounds, arms, and feet until you complete your walk.

Step Four: Celebrate that you practiced mindfulness today.

Stress-Management Promise

Please follow the schedule in this section.

Swap days around depending on work/school/life, and, of course, practice any self-management practices you already enjoy.

Every day this week, I promise to:

• Practice self-compassion whenever negative, judgmental, or painful thoughts arise. Revisit page 92 for a refresher.

• Choose one thing each day in which I am fully present and practice mindfulness (washing the dishes, brushing my teeth, cooking dinner, etc.).

Monday: Twenty minutes of solitude (no texts, podcasts, music, or media of any kind).

Tuesday: Mindful walking or meditation of your choice.

Wednesday: Practice grounding for five minutes (close your eyes, feel the weight of your feet on the ground, your bottom in the chair, your body in the bed, etc.).

Thursday: Twenty minutes of solitude (no texts, podcasts, music, or media of any kind).

Friday: Mindful walking or meditation of your choice.

Saturday: Find and put into motion your new stress-management hobby: buy a puzzle, bust out (or get new) art supplies, find a crocheting/knitting tutorial online, start a window garden, and/or think about the hobbies you loved as a kid and try one again.

Sunday: One full day of no social media. If you aren't on social, sub with two twenty-minute rounds of solitude (one in the morning and one at night).

Week Three: Good Food

There are no rules, laws or traditions that apply universally . . .
including this one.

—WAYNE DYER

Defining what makes up "the endo diet" feels like an impossible task. There are so many different variations and versions of it out there that it's hard to know which one to follow. Some versions are cool with caffeine, and some think it's the devil. Some include eggs, while others say "never!" Some say grains should never be on your plate, while others say they're fine (just as long as they're gluten-free). This is in addition to the hundreds of nutrition experts and influencers confusing us even more with their own diet dos and don'ts that have nothing to do with endo. Someone over here tells you that you *need* to eat meat to be healthy, while someone over there tells you that vegan is the only way to go. Some days coconut oil is good. But wait, now it's bad! It can feel impossible to keep up and know what to eat.

And now here I am, yet another person who's going to tell you what to eat and confuse you more. Except that's not what I'm going to do. I'm not able to tell you the exact right thing to eat for your body, because I'm not in your body. But what I can do is help guide you to discover the best foods for *you*. There is not one endo diet for everyone. Just like that Wayne Dyer quote, there are no rules or laws that universally apply here. It's about finding *your* good foods.

I've experimented a lot over the years, and after a lot of trial and error, I was able to develop a good foods foundation that works for me. I was able to identify my food triggers (the foods that make my endo happy or mad) and alter my diet as I went. This foundation has changed my entire life, and I want to help you build your new foundation, too— a foundation that will allow for change and gives you the freedom to experiment to find **your good foods.**

From this point forward, we're ditching the term "endo diet" and focusing on good foods.

Good foods are:
1. Foods that nourish and energize you.
2. Foods that don't hurt you and/or make your endo symptoms feel worse.

Good foods are *not:*
A restrictive diet, steamed broccoli and rice for every meal, a static plan that can never change, the magic solution to getting skinny, a cure for endo, or a universal standard.

It's also not about labels. Our culture loves labels when it comes to food and diets! I get it. Labels can help us streamline the process of change, make it easier to find recipes and cookbooks that align with our new diet and lifestyle, and connect us to like-minded communities that eat the same as we do. But they can also feel limiting and intimidating. Most of us have had that feeling of "failing" after trying a new diet and eating one of that diet's "forbidden" foods. It can send you into a shame spiral of stress, which—as we've already learned—is not good for our endo. It can also cause a lot of anxiety if you've had a history of disordered eating. Creating this new foundation and finding your good foods is not about labels, and it's not about being perfect. It's about adding more foods to your diet that make you feel good—and less of the ones that make you feel bad.

I think it's important to mention that after you find the foods that make you feel good, you might still decide to eat foods that make you feel not so good. I eat big piles of fries from time to time and have a hard time saying no to a tub of hummus (it's one of my number-one bloat-inducing foods, and one that I know I need to eat in moderation). I know these things might not make me feel my best after I eat them, but that doesn't make me or the food *bad*. Finding your good foods is not about villainizing categories of foods or never eating them again. It's about empowering yourself to have more control over how you feel. Whether you choose to eat your good foods 100 percent of the time or 50 percent of the time is entirely up to you.

Once we can all get on board with the fact that there is no one perfect endo diet for everyone, it becomes so much easier to shut out the noise of what everyone else is eating and focus solely on you. Finding your good foods can be incredibly powerful and life changing, but it can get a little complicated, too. It's rare that someone will master this tool all in one week. It's usually not as simple as a quick trip to the grocery store and POOF!, you magically know the perfect foods for your body. And unless you're Oprah status and have a personal chef preparing every meal for you, *you* have to make a choice as to what those meals are. It can feel overwhelming at first. It takes time not only to figure out the best foods for your body but also to work through the emotional and social challenges this tool can bring, too.

Okay, so what emotional and social challenges are we talking about here?

Well, for most of our lives, we've created traditions, rituals, stories, and habits around food—some that were passed down to us through generations of our families and some that we've created on our own.

What is your greatest endo management tool?

Food and self-compassion! Changing what I put into my body was a game changer for my endo symptoms.

—Sherilynn Sherrouse

These rituals and traditions can feel so familiar and like such an integral part of our lives that we might not even realize how much they inform our food identity. We use food, with our family and friends, as a way to celebrate our successes, holidays, and biggest life events. And for many of us, we also use food as a way to comfort ourselves when we're sad, anxious, and even bored. It can feel scary and uncomfortable to change these food traditions and habits, not just for us but also for the people in our lives who have shared these traditions with us over the years. These habits and traditions will definitely play a major role in how you approach this week's tool. Will I be asking you to ditch all of these special traditions and habits? No way. But I will ask you to challenge which ones make you and your endo feel best and to think about tweaks to them to help you feel better.

Doctors + Diet

Changing my diet was one of the hardest things I've ever done. I was not that rare person who mastered it in one week, and I'm definitely not Oprah status with a chef cooking all my meals. Granted, back then I didn't really cook for myself, either. And if I was going to cook, I for sure wasn't going to cook vegetables. I liked easy, convenient food. I really do mean convenient food—foods that you can get at the convenience store. Foods that had half-decade-long expiration dates, made with impossible-to-pronounce ingredients, and/or could easily be microwaved. I like to joke that my favorite food groups used to be: Gummy Candies, Diet Coke, and Whatever Frozen Meal Had the Most Cheese. These were my comfort foods, and because I was in so much pain, I wanted to be comforted all the time.

The wild thing is that I didn't even realize that these foods were making my pain feel worse. Even wilder, not one single doctor in the marathon of doctors I saw ever once asked me about my diet. Which is not entirely their fault. Most doctors are simply not taught enough about nutrition in medical school. A report by the *Journal of Biomedical Education* found that 86 of the 121 US medical schools that participated in the report failed to provide the recommended minimum twenty-five hours of nutrition education; forty-three provided less than half that much.[1]

In addition to the lack of education, most doctors need data and definitive research to even consider suggesting something to a patient. And we're not there yet when it comes to the data and research about endometriosis and diet. At a recent appointment with a new ob-gyn, she asked how I was managing my endometriosis if I wasn't on the pill or other hormonal treatments. I told her that my low-inflammatory diet was my biggest management tool. She smirked, said she had never heard that one before, and asked if I had any studies to back it up. I politely told her she could go online and search "endo" and "diet" to explore it herself. But even if I had thought to come prepared with printouts proving my case, there really isn't anything to print out. At the time of writing this book, there still aren't any big peer-reviewed studies that prove that diet can help endometriosis. The studies I did find (some of which were performed on rats) ended with statements such as "No clear recommendations on what diet to eat or refrain from to reduce the symptoms of endometriosis can be given." And, "Evidence supporting a role of diet on endometriosis risk is equivocal."[2,3]

Yes, there are doctors who believe in the power of good food and its connection to endo, but they seem to be rare. I hear from friendos all the time who say their doctors tell them diet will have no impact on their endo symptoms and pain. One woman told me that she was laughed at and made to feel stupid for even bringing it up to her doctor. I once proudly told a doctor I knew at a conference how much diet has changed my life. This wasn't just any doctor—he's a pretty famous one who wrote one of the most well-known books on the positive impact of diet on chronic illness. He congratulated me but quickly added that my story was merely anecdotal and there are no conclusive studies to prove that diet can help endometriosis. I know, buddy. I know.

But here's the thing. I don't need the studies. I have conducted my own little study over the last decade, and I have all the conclusive answers I need. My good foods have changed my life, and I've witnessed them help countless other people with endo, too. There might not be conclusive research on the impact of diet on endo (yet), but there are plenty of studies and books that show the powerful and profound impact that a low-inflammatory diet can have on our bodies. And if endometriosis is, at its core, an inflammatory condition, wouldn't a diet rich in low-inflammatory foods be helpful? Wouldn't cutting back on inflammatory foods potentially help a body that is chronically inflamed? I don't need big studies to understand the basic logic of this.

So, Let's Talk Inflammation

As we've discussed, you'll be hard-pressed to find a single diet theory that everyone can agree on. But one idea remains pretty consistent in every camp: inflammatory foods are not our friends, especially for people with inflammatory conditions. I spoke with gastroenterologist and gut health expert Dr. Will Bulsiewicz (Dr. B) about this, and he explained that there are two types of inflammation: acute and chronic. Acute is the inflammatory or immune response to an acute stressor (a surgery, trauma, or an infection). Chronic inflammation is the low-level ongoing activation of the immune system. I asked him if he would consider people with endometriosis as having chronic inflammation, and he said, "One hundred percent, they're living with chronic inflammation."

So, what happens when you're living with chronic inflammation and then you add inflammatory foods on top of it? It's like adding fuel to your chronic-inflammation fire. As we learned in Chapter 2, GI issues are one of the first symptoms that the majority of people present to their doctors, and the big inflammatory foods might be making them worse.

What Are the Big Inflammatories (BI)?

The main culprits include:
Processed and packaged foods

Dairy products (milk, cheese, yogurt)

Red meat

Refined sugars + synthetic sweeteners

Fried foods

Soda

Refined carbohydrates (cookies, cakes, pretzels, etc.)

Alcohol

Caffeine

Some people also experience increased symptoms from eating eggs, grains, corn, and nightshade vegetables (eggplant, peppers, tomatoes, and potatoes). These aren't necessarily foods that cause inflammation for us all, but foods that we can have sensitivities to and our gut has a hard time processing, which can result in digestive issues (bloating, gas, and stomach pain).

So, what the heck are you supposed to eat? I know. You may have seen some of your favorite foods in the list above, and that's okay. Don't worry about that right now. I'm not going to say you can never eat them again and ask you to cut every single one out. There might be some that you can tolerate just fine. But as you begin to build your good foods foundation, it's important to be aware of the biggest culprits.

Building a Good Foods Foundation

Like I said, your good foods might be different from mine, but we all need a good foundation to begin. This week, our foundation will be focused on low-inflammatory, plant-heavy whole foods. Which sounds like a lot of things! It also sounds "label-y" when I just said I don't like labels. But stay with me. You never have to use these terms to describe your diet if someone asks. You can simply tell them that you're focused on eating good foods that don't make you feel bad (or actually, you don't have to explain yourself at all). I'm using these words not as labels but to give you a clear picture of the foods we'll be focusing on this week—and to help you navigate your cupboards and the grocery store as you build your foundation.

So, let's break down what these phrases mean.

Low-inflammatory

I like to use the term "low-inflammatory" instead of the more common term "anti-inflammatory." With endo, we'll never be able to completely get rid of our inflammation with food, so "anti" is a little misleading. Dr. B explains, "There is no such thing as no inflammation." He says to think of inflammation like a stereo system. You can have the music blasting so loud that it hurts your ears *or* you can have the music quiet and peaceful. Because there will always be inflammation, it's about making sure that it's not being disruptive and causing issues. It's focusing on the foods that you can rely on your gut to process and digest.

So, how do we start eating a low-inflammatory diet? The answer is simple: start making plant-heavy whole-food meals (we'll talk about those next) that don't include (or limit) foods in our BI list. I understand that it's never fun to focus on all the things you can't eat, but it's also really important to be aware of the foods that might be increasing your inflammation and digestive issues. Focusing on reducing and eliminating the foods on this list is not a new diet trend to help you get rid of some weight. This is a new way of eating to help you limit your pain and symptoms.

This is a huge difference in perspective, and it might require a mindset shift to think of food in this way. If you've come from a place of chronic dieting or disordered eating, it's understandable that it might be hard to eat for your health and not for your weight. Jessica Duffin, a certified women's health coach specializing in endometriosis, shares that a lot of people who want to change their diet aren't ready to take out whole categories of food, or they feel anxiety around the word "elimination," so she suggests not to think about taking foods out but rather "crowding" in new ones. Working with a coach like Jessica—or a nutritionist who specializes in disordered eating—can be incredibly valuable if you're struggling with making this change.

It's also important to remember that you don't have to be perfect or all-or-nothing to begin. For instance, when I first started changing my diet, I limited dairy to once a week. Was it easy? No. I cried about it for the first two months. I felt really angry that my endo was interfering with yet another thing in my life (my love of cheese). But after a while, I noticed that on the days I had dairy, I didn't feel so great. So those dairy days became once a month or on special occasions. And then those days didn't feel worth it anymore, either. Today I'm almost a decade in without dairy, something I never thought I would or could do! My pain and symptoms are so much better now that I don't cry over cheese. Not to mention, I've found some amazing substitutions that are just as good.

You are the only one who knows how your body feels when you eat certain foods, and it's your responsibility to listen to it. It's a process to learn how to communicate with your body and to understand what it's trying to tell you, but my guess is that it's giving you some cues already. Do you feel more bloated or have painful bowel movements after eating a lot of baked goods? After eating a lot of sugar, do you feel sad, moody, fatigued, or more anxious? Do your joints feel sore and achy after a cheese platter, or maybe you're constipated?

Sometimes these cues are subtle hints, and sometimes they're being shouted at you loud and clear. Either way, we usually don't *want* to really hear what our bodies are saying. It never feels good admitting that something we really love makes us feel really bad. So, it's okay if you're not ready to give up everything at once. But you must at least start to notice these cues and get really honest with yourself about how certain foods make you feel. This information will be your guide, whether you go all in now or decide to go slow and steady with your changes.

Plant-Heavy Whole Foods

"Plant-heavy" means a focus on veggies, fruits, grains, nuts, seeds, and legumes, with little to no animal products (dairy, meat, and eggs). I won't be asking you to go vegan, but I will be asking you to introduce one or two completely plant-based meals a day that do not include the BIs or animal products. You'll also notice that none of the recipes in this book have animal products in them. Why? Many people with endo experience increased symptoms when eating eggs, dairy gives them digestive issues, and they just feel better after removing meat. But you might not know if you're one of these people until you try leaving them off your plate.

When I changed my diet, I hung on to eggs for dear life, because they were easy, and I knew I could always get them at a restaurant. But after I slowly started eliminating the BIs (no more bread, cheese, and bacon that I usually ate with my eggs), I was left with simple scrambled eggs. By eating the eggs all alone, I soon became aware that they were a huge digestive trigger for me. After eliminating them and reintroducing them, you may realize that eggs are just fine for you. But you also might realize that they play a role in impacting your symptoms and/or pain. You just won't know until you try.

Excluding animal products from your diet can feel difficult at first, especially when it comes to eating out or traveling. It's not uncommon to see a menu that has steak, chicken, or fish as the only protein options, but there are ways to make it work. Later in this chapter, I'll give you some tips to make it easier.

Whole Foods

"Whole foods" mean foods that are minimally processed—or not processed at all—and free of additives and artificial ingredients. This doesn't mean that you can never buy something that is processed ever again. In fact, you'll see a few minimally processed ingredients in the recipes ahead (rice pasta and almond butter, for example). But it does mean getting really good at reading labels at the grocery store and being more conscious about what's in your food. For example, one of the most popular "maple syrup" brands doesn't even contain maple syrup. Check out the ingredient list: *high-fructose corn syrup, corn syrup, water, salt, cellulose gum, molasses, potassium sorbate (preservative), sodium hexametaphosphate, citric acid, caramel color, natural and artificial flavors.* No maple syrup! The whole-food version would include one ingredient: maple syrup. Another example is peanut butter. Most big-name peanut butter brands include sugar and hydrogenated vegetable or soybean oils. You might be thinking that there's no way that your peanut butter has sugar in it. But flip over that label and check for yourself. You'd be surprised that it is the second ingredient in most big-name peanut butter brands, even the "natural" ones. When you're shopping for peanut or nut butters, look for ones that have the nuts and some salt (and that's it!).

Not every single thing you put in your grocery cart needs to be in its whole form and contain fewer than three ingredients, but at least start to look and become more aware of what those ingredients are. In the beginning, it can definitely make your shopping trips longer and may even cause a little anxiety that you aren't "doing it right." I know this was true for me. The thing that helped my shopping anxiety the most was creating a Top Ten pantry list. These were the ten items whose ingredients I knew by heart, were staples for my recipes, and, most important, made me feel good—things like tahini, some grains and seeds, and coconut milk. This made shopping feel way less stressful, and I knew that if I had my Top Ten and some veggies, I could whip something up fast for dinner. If you want to learn more about this, my cookbook, *One Part Plant*, goes more in-depth into the specifics of my Top Ten, where to find them at the store, and label reading, too.

Questions?

Whenever I talk about a plant-heavy whole-food diet, I can count on the same questions/comments to come up every time. They're some of the same questions and thoughts I had when I first started discovering my good foods, so I totally understand where they're coming from. *One Part Plant* also covers these questions more in depth, but I wanted to make sure to give you an abridged version here.

How Will I Get My Protein if I Am Cutting Out or Limiting Animal Products?

I always think it's funny when people ask me if I'm getting enough protein, because no one ever asked me that when I was eating meat. Most people don't even know how much protein we're supposed to consume each day, but they become very concerned about that amount when you start eating more plants. The simple answer is: you will get all the protein you need with a well-rounded, whole-food, plant-heavy diet that is full of beans, lentils, grains, nuts, seeds, and veggies (yes, some veggies have protein!). And an added bonus of plant-based proteins is that you get all the benefits without the cholesterol and potential hormones found in animal-sourced proteins.

If you're still concerned about how much protein you need, or feel like you need to amp it up because you are an athlete, you can find protein calculators online to help you with the recommended amount for your body weight and activity level. There are a lot of high-performing body builders, ultra-marathon runners, mixed martial arts athletes, and tennis and basketball players who are 100 percent plant-based, and you can check them out to help reassure you that you can still perform at your best with only plants.

It Sounds Expensive to Eat This Way!
It can be, but it doesn't have to be. Eating more plants doesn't mean you have to buy $25 jars of almond butter or pricey, artisanal, dairy-free cheese. If you can afford them, cool. If not, it isn't a deal breaker. It's really fun to explore all of the specialty plant-based food brands out there, but I like to think of these as fun/special treats—and not part of my Top Ten.

Shopping in the bulk section for nuts, seeds, and grains can save you a lot of money, and so does buying frozen fruits and veggies (especially when they aren't in season). It's also important to point out that a pound of lentils is way less expensive than a pound of grass-fed/organic meat— because if you are going to eat meat, it's important to buy organic and/ or grass-fed, which doesn't include the hormones and antibiotics that factory-farmed meat generally has. Not everyone can afford or has access to grass-fed/organic meats, which might make the decision to eat a plant-heavy diet even easier.

Speaking of organic, I know there a lot of wellness gurus out there saying that you must buy all your produce organic. It would be amazing if we could all do that, but that's just not possible for everyone when it comes to availability and/or our budgets. Just do your best when it comes to buying your produce, and buy organic when you can. The Environmental Working Group's Clean Fifteen and Dirty Dozen Lists are great guides to shopping organic. These lists come out every year and include the fruits and veggies with the least and most amounts of pesticides. For instance, this year, avocado and pineapple are at the top of the Clean Fifteen, and strawberries and spinach are at the top of the Dirty Dozen. So, if you're only able to shop for some organic things, go for the organic strawberries and spinach and go conventional for the avocados and pineapple. You can also peel the fruits and/or vegetables (cucumbers, apples, pears, and potatoes) if they are not organic, which helps, too.

I Don't Have Time to Eat This Way or I Don't Know How to Cook

Whenever someone tells me that they don't have time to eat whole-food, plant-heavy meals, I ask them what types of dishes they think they have to make. Yes, dehydrating beets for twelve hours and making your own fermented raw cashew cheese would take a long time, but so does cooking a pot roast and making homemade croissants. If you like complicated and more time-intensive recipes, go for it! But if you're short on time or don't love spending a lot of time in the kitchen, choose easy, thirty-minute-or-less recipes the same way you would if you were making non-plant-heavy meals (I'll be sharing some of my favorites in the recipe section of this chapter).

If you truly don't have time to cook or shop, there is nothing wrong with plant-heavy whole-food prepared meal delivery, meal kits, ordering in, or getting takeout. Just be mindful of how the food is prepared and ask questions if you're not sure. I remember once ordering baba ghanoush from a new Mediterranean restaurant in my neighborhood and having horrible GI issues after eating it. Baba ghanoush wasn't something that bothered me before, so I called the restaurant to ask the ingredients and learned they used yogurt in their recipe to make it creamier. I hadn't had this dish with added dairy before, so it wasn't something I thought to ask, but now I always do. It might feel uncomfortable to ask these types of questions at first, but those few minutes of feeling uncomfortable are worth it to avoid eating something that could make you uncomfortable for hours.

And in terms of not cooking . . . I have a hard time giving anyone a pass on this one. Because I never cooked before, either. Remember, my main food groups used to be gummy worms and microwavable meals. I was pretty scared of the kitchen and felt like cooking would never be something I could be good at. But just like most things in our lives, we have to practice in order to get better. For me, it took changing my mind-set about cooking. I wasn't just trying to cook to get better at it—I was trying to cook to feel better. Because I understand what it's like to have zero confidence in the kitchen, my advice is not to start with a recipe that requires twenty ingredients and lots of steps. Choose recipes that are easy and require a handful of ingredients. You might not master a complicated gluten-free tiramisu right now, but maybe you make the best three-ingredient, no-bake cookies anyone has ever had. Cooking classes (virtual or in-person) are also a great way to gain more confidence in the kitchen.

Keep in mind, cooking doesn't always have to be this precious, romantic, and mindful process all the time. It can be, but it can also be streaming your favorite show or podcast in the background or multitasking by talking to a friend while you cook. Do whatever works to get yourself in the kitchen and eating your good food meals. Practice, burn stuff, and get better as you go.

Do I Need to Be Gluten-Free?

Oh, "the glutes," as we lovingly call it in my house. There are so many new theories and books out every year about whether we should or shouldn't eat gluten that it's made us all terrified to eat a piece of toast. I asked Dr. B to break it down for us. He says there are three major groups of people who should not be eating gluten. Those are people with (1) celiac disease; (2) a wheat allergy; and (3) non-celiac gluten sensitivity with extraintestinal symptoms.

So, if It's Only These Three Groups That Shouldn't Be Eating Gluten, Then Why Does Gluten Make a Lot of Us Feel So Bad Most of the Time?

Dr. B says that most foods that have gluten are "highly processed foods" (baked goods and snack foods). So when you feel bad after eating these foods, you have to ask yourself if it's the gluten causing the problem or the other ingredients. And is it only gluten-containing processed foods, or is it processed foods, period?

Okay, So We Should Just Buy Gluten-Free Products, Then?

Not exactly. Dr. B says that when it comes to gluten-free products on the market, "Ninety-five percent of what's out there is trash. It used to be that ten years ago, if you went gluten-free, you're eating a pretty damn clean diet because gluten-free packaged foods did not exist." But that all changed when the gluten-free diet craze began and the gluten-free food industry boomed because of public demand. Now, gluten-free packaged foods can make you feel just as bad as the ones you were trying to eliminate in the first place.

Where Does This Leave Us?

If you have celiac disease, a wheat allergy, or a non-celiac gluten sensitivity with extraintestinal symptoms, do not eat gluten moving forward. But if you're like the rest of us, you can experiment to see how gluten makes you feel. *But let's be clear.* This doesn't mean testing your tolerance for gluten with a giant slice of pizza, a box of doughnuts, or other processed foods. We're talking about whole grains, a good sourdough bread, and/or a sprouted one like Ezekiel bread. This could also mean eating grains that are naturally gluten-free, too, like buckwheat, amaranth, millet, oats, and rice.

Personally, I've found that I can tolerate some sourdough and sprouted breads, and I eat them on occasion. But I avoid them during the days leading up to and during my period. They can be harder for me to digest, and I like to give my stomach a break during those days. I've also found that brown rice is hard for me to digest at times, so I eat it in very small amounts or stick to quinoa, gluten-free oats, and millet. You'll need to find what works for you, but the first step is removing the packaged/processed gluten-containing foods in your diet and replacing them with whole foods.

What about Coffee and Alcohol?

I remember a woman in one of my Know Your Endo course sessions who removed coffee from her routine and was amazed at just how much it was contributing to her pain and symptoms. She felt so much better without it. But then another student said she didn't notice a difference at all by removing it. This is an example of how everyone's endo and bodies will react differently to different things. Jessica Duffin says that studies have shown that caffeine can increase inflammation in some people and elevate cortisol, which can wreak havoc on your hormones. She notes that it can also aggravate GI symptoms and increase feelings of anxiety—things that people with endo might already be experiencing—so it's worth eliminating it for a couple of weeks to see if caffeine is impacting your body.

I'm not saying this is an easy task! So many people rely on coffee to start their day, and the act of making a cup and sitting down to drink it has become a sacred ritual in their lives. As I said earlier, I'm not asking you to give up the habits you love, but you might need to tweak them to feel better. This might mean limiting the amount of coffee you drink, replacing your cream with a nut milk, ditching the sweetener, and/or replacing your coffee with an herbal-blend alternative. Will these alternatives taste exactly like the coffee you're drinking right now? No. But they can come close and provide a way to maintain the morning habit and ritual so many of us crave.

In terms of alcohol, most of us already know that alcohol is an inflammatory for our bodies and can have various other unhealthy side effects. If you've ever had a massive hangover, then you've already experienced what your body thought about the drinks you consumed the night before. These body cues are usually pretty obvious—you have a lot of drinks at your friend's birthday party and the next day you have a pounding headache, feel sick, and just want to lie in bed all day. But what might not be so obvious is the impact that alcohol has on your pain and endo symptoms. And this is incredibly important to track. Start tuning in to your body and endo symptoms after you drink. For example, after a week of work dinners packed with cocktails and more after-dinner drinks, how do your period cramps feel? What about your fatigue the next day after a few glasses of wine? How is your digestion after that second round of beers?

Drinking can make us more relaxed in social situations and is a way to celebrate with friends. But once you start listening to what your body has to say about drinking, and if it's telling you, *"Yeah, not so much,"* it might be time to switch it up. This could mean replacing three super-sugary margaritas with one good sipping tequila with lime—or having one glass of wine instead of sharing a whole bottle with a friend. After experimenting with what works for you, you might learn that you need to eliminate alcohol altogether.

If you decide to limit your drinking or eliminate it completely, it can definitely be a challenge in social situations. Sometimes we just say yes to the glass of wine because we want to avoid all the questions that arise if we say no. *Why aren't you drinking? Are you pregnant? Boooo! Don't you want to have fun?* Ruby Warrington's book *Sober Curious* is an incredible resource to help guide you through these tricky social situations and help you explore your relationship with alcohol in a nonjudgmental (and realistic) way.

I had the opportunity to interview Ruby about her book and the sober curious movement during her book tour, and she said something in that interview that I'll never forget. She said that when we use alcohol "to dim the darkness, we can also dim the light." We might drink to try to manage or dim the dark parts we don't want to face (our social anxieties, our pain, or a horrible day at work), but we can't control if that alcohol is also dimming the light parts, too (our joy, creativity, and things we're passionate about). We don't get to decide what alcohol will choose to dim, and you have to decide when or if you're okay with this or not.

Listening to your body and reading up on the sober curious movement can be helpful if you're a casual to moderate drinker, but if you're using alcohol as a daily coping mechanism, these tools might not be enough. Research shows that as many as 28 percent of people with chronic pain use alcohol to try to cope with and alleviate their pain. And according to the National Institute on Alcohol Abuse and Alcoholism, "Withdrawal from chronic alcohol use often increases pain sensitivity which could motivate some people to continue drinking or even increase their drinking to reverse withdrawal-related increases in pain."[4] This can be yet another vicious cycle that endo can create. If you know that you are using alcohol or drugs to manage the physical and mental toll of endo and want to stop but find that your pain is worse every time you do, I urge you to seek help. Talk to your doctor, a professional counselor, or a friend to help you seek resources in your area that can help.

Is Soy Really Bad for You?

Soy is another tricky one, like gluten. There are studies to support both sides of the spectrum (it being good or bad for our bodies), and some people find that they are more sensitive to it than others. And just like gluten, there are a lot of genetically modified and processed soy products out there (ice cream, burgers, etc.), and it's a filler ingredient in a lot of packaged foods. It's a good idea to stay away from the soy-filled processed foods and stick to organic and non-GMO varieties of tempeh, edamame, miso, tofu, and tamari (a gluten-free soy sauce) in moderation. Track how you feel when consuming these products to determine how they impact you.

And What about Sugar?

Sugar is one of the biggest inflammatories for our bodies, but it's also one that is sometimes the hardest to let go of—because it's in every-thing! From pasta sauces to peanut butter, it's a big ingredient found in a lot of packaged foods (and foods where you'd least expect it). As you begin to limit and eliminate the BIs, it's important to keep in mind that sugar is sugar, whether the bag just says "sugar" or "organic evaporated cane juice."

Jessica Duffin, who we heard from earlier in this chapter, shares that even high-sugar fruits can affect us. She shared from her own experi-ence that if she eats high-sugar fruits before or during her period, she notices that her pain shoots up. She told me, "I could have a mango and it's game over." This doesn't mean you can never have a mango again. It just means you have to remember to tap into how higher-sugar fruits make you feel during different parts of the month. You may find that they don't affect you at all, or that they're a trigger for you.

In the recipes ahead, you'll see that I use natural sweeteners such as dates, maple syrup, and raw honey. Yes, these are still sugars. And yes, we still need to be aware of how they make us feel. But in moderation, they can help make this transition easier. It did for me. Candy, cook-ies, and cakes were a big part of my life before I changed my diet. Not just because I loved the taste of them, but because they were a part of traditions I had with my family and friends—making cookies at Christ-mas, celebrating with giant cakes at birthday parties, and sharing pints of ice cream while watching movies together.

When I changed my diet, I really thought I'd have to say goodbye to all of these traditions and shared experiences with food, and I was pretty emotional about it. After feeling sad for a couple of months, I decided to do something about it and began to teach myself how to make some of those sweet treats in a way that would work for me. I used maple syrup in place of white sugar. I used dates to make plant-based caramel. After a lot of trial and error, I came up with treats that didn't hurt my endo. I don't eat these things all the time, but knowing that I can has helped me so much, and I'm hoping it helps you, too.

Am I perfect about sugar? No. If I'm at a party and someone hands me a slice of vegan cake, I'm most likely gonna eat it. The difference now is that I'm much more mindful about how that sugar makes me feel, and I can make more conscious choices about when and when not to eat it. For example, if I'm on my period or it's days away, that cake is going to land me in bed (or on the toilet in pain). So on those days, I'd pass on the cake at the party and bring my own dessert, which we'll talk about more in a minute.

What's your ideal relationship with endo?

A place of balance.

—Alaia Baldwin Aronow

Do I Really Have to Drink a Ton of Water?
Yes, please. Most of us know that water can help with digestion, better skin, and, well, we need it to survive (pretty big one). But it can also help with our brain health. Studies show that even mild dehydration can cause brain fog, mood swings, and headaches.[5] This is huge, especially if you're already dealing with fatigue, brain fog, and mood swings from your endo!

I've never been great at drinking enough water. I'd tell myself that I'd answer one more email and then get water. That turned into twenty emails, fixing dinner, doing laundry, and going to bed grouchy with a headache before realizing I had only had about a shot glass full of water all day (and that was to take my vitamins). I *need* reminders, accountability, and goals. So, I have a piece of paper stuck to my fridge with the word "water" typed out and the days of the week next to it. I strive to drink four big mason jars a day, and when I drink all my water for the day, I get to fill in the box. I get so much pleasure coloring in that box at the end of the day, and I'm not sure I'd be drinking as much without it. Other water tips: set a timer for each hour you're awake and drink a glass each time the alarm goes off, or have a giant jug of water that you must finish by the end of the day. There are even water tracking apps to send you reminders. Do whatever you need to do to get your water in each day!

How Do I Eat This Way with Family/Out with Friends/Traveling?
In the first decade of my marriage, my husband would make big bowls of sautéed greens with rice and beans, while I opted for big bowls of Lucky Charms and ice cream. While he never pressured me to eat the foods he was eating, deep down I was a little jealous of the way he ate. That jealousy came out by way of judging, turning my nose up at his dishes, and then rebelling by giving myself another scoop of ice cream.

Today we share those bowls of rice and beans (and I actually like greens). But I had to find my good foods and understand the power of plant-heavy whole foods on my own. As you begin to change your diet and get in tune with what your body needs over the next few months, it might surprise you that not everyone will be on board with this change. You might get a lot of questions, concerns, and pushback from your family and friends. They might be clinging to their own version of Lucky Charms and ice cream and don't want to hear about your new food ways and how good you feel. They might feel hurt that you are changing traditions you shared together. They might even feel a little jealous that you are making a change that they always wanted to make themselves. Like I said, this is a complicated tool. But after nearly a decade navigating these changes, I can tell you that it gets easier (and more fun).

1. Ease into It (Together).
Cooking for yourself is one thing, but if you're responsible for cooking meals for your kids, spouse, or really any family member who lives with you, it can be tricky at first. You want to respect that not everyone is choosing to change their diet with you, but you also don't want to make two different meals every night for dinner. The solution is to ease them into your new good foods while still honoring their favorites, too.

- **Make food they love without labels.**

  This might sound obvious, but sometimes we get so excited about how our new diet is making us feel that we go overboard with the details and it can turn some people off. As my good friend DeMar always says, "If there was a giant VEGAN sign above the produce section in the grocery store, no one would ever buy an apple again." So, on the night you serve lasagna (Creamy Roasted Broccoli + Swiss Chard Lasagna, page 163), there's no need to talk about how dairy-free, gluten-free, and plant-based it is. Just serve it! After everyone has cleaned their plates and asked for seconds, you can always share how that meal is part of your new good foods, and that you're so excited to make more of these recipes to enjoy together.

- **Add toppers!**

  If your family cannot fathom not adding cheese to their rice and beans or think you've lost your mind omitting beef from their beloved spaghetti sauce, you can still create one base meal for the table. Your base recipe will incorporate your good foods, and the rest will be toppers your family can add themselves—which might mean stirring their own beef into a sauce and/or adding their own cheese. There are also a lot of great meat substitutes and dairy alternatives that you can use as you transition together, too.

- **Take it slow.**

  You cannot expect you and your family to go from zero to green smoothies in one week. It will take time and a little trial and error to find what works. The only thing you can do is lead by example and do your best to make good foods they love. Taste buds will change, resistance will fade, and you'll eventually find your new good-foods groove, together.

2. Always Choose the Restaurant.

When you are going out to dinner with family or friends or having a business lunch with a client, jump in and choose the restaurant first. This doesn't mean choosing a spot that only serves your diet needs. It's choosing one where you know you can find an option—and everyone else can, too.

3. Be Prepared at Parties/Celebrations/Holidays.

There is no guarantee there will be something you can eat at gatherings with friends and family—I cannot stress this enough. Try it and see what happens. Actually, don't try it. Because chances are, you'll end up holding a plate with just a few carrot sticks, and maybe some celery. Always bring a dish to share that you know you can eat (this is especially important for big holidays).

- **BYOD (Bring Your Own Dessert).**
  At events where you can't bring a dish to eat, like a wedding, you can usually request a special meal for yourself. It's not likely that you'll also be able to request a special dessert, so bring your own! Whenever I go to weddings, I stash my own dessert in my bag and pull it out when they serve the cake. Yes, I could live a little and just eat the wedding cake. But over time, I realized it's just not worth it anymore. It isn't worth the risk of that cake making me feel super bloated and sending me straight to the bathroom (instead of the dance floor). BYOD whenever you can.

- **Create Swaps and New Traditions.**
  Instead of banishing your grandma's mashed potatoes at Thanksgiving forever, could you swap nondairy milk and butter for her traditional butter and cream? Or instead of celebrating your birthday every year with pizza and beer, could you create a tradition

that incorporates your new good foods (foods that still feel fun and celebratory but don't make you feel bad)? You don't have to abandon all of the food traditions you love. You just might need to create some new ones.

- **Have Something, *Anything* on Your Plate.**
  The times I've gotten the most questions and concerns about my diet is when I have an empty plate at a party or holiday celebration. An empty plate will not only draw attention, it can potentially hurt your host's feelings. (*Did she not like the food? I feel so bad she can't eat anything! I'm such a bad host.*) I don't want my food choices to make anyone ever feel bad or be the focus of the meal. Just another reason to always bring a dish you can eat and share.

4. Plan Ahead When You Travel.

When flying, I always make sure to have two to three snacks in my bag, in case of emergencies. This is usually an apple, a sleeve of almond butter, and some sort of bar. I've even traveled with an avocado and a fork before (when I knew there were going to be zero options at the airport).

When you get to your destination, do a little shopping. Find a store nearby that has packaged meals and more snacks (again, in case of emergencies). Sometimes that means venturing a little outside your comfort zone to find what you need. When I first changed my diet, I'd always look for the old-school hippie health shop in whatever city I was in. This wasn't really in my comfort zone, but they always had something for me to eat, so I kept it up. Now it feels like an adventure to find these shops, and it's become one of my favorite parts of a trip.

You can also scope out the restaurants in advance, especially on road trips. Have a few places planned so you don't panic when you're starving and eat something that doesn't make you feel awesome. And if you know there isn't going to be any place to stop on your five-hour drive, bring your own food. I understand that stopping along the way at roadside diners is part of the road-trip experience, but wouldn't you rather feel good when you reach your destination than have a belly full of food that doesn't make you feel your best?

———

While all of these tricks and tips are ones that are setting you up for success, sometimes you'll still find resistance from your family and friends. This might require a little sit-down discussion to let them know just how important this change is to you. This is not a fad diet or something you're trying to do for a month to get skinny. This is something you plan on doing long-term, because you want to enjoy your life more with them and not be in pain. You're not asking for a standing ovation every time you drink a smoothie, but you do want their support in your pursuit to feel better.

Ready?

Before you head over to your Good Foods Promise this week, there are a few things I need for you to keep in mind before you get started.

1. You'll see that your promise is only one week long, but please do not stop there. This isn't a cleanse where you are taking out everything for a week and then going back to your normal food routine. You are building new, sustainable habits that will last your lifetime.

    Please give your body the opportunity to eat plant-heavy whole-food meals for at least thirty days . . . and go from there. These changes will take time for your body and brain to adjust to. If you have work or family events, a vacation, or just a stressful day that throws you off your game, jump right back in as soon as you can. You might not do these perfectly, and that's okay. Like I said, this is not a cleanse. You have thousands of meals ahead of you. You don't need to get every single one perfect.

2. In the following pages, I've included a handful of recipes to give you inspiration and help you get started. I'm hoping some of them become staples in your kitchen, but this is not a set meal plan. You don't *have* to eat these specifically to succeed. Feel free to change them up to suit your body's needs and dietary preferences, and riff on them to create your own version of the dish. At knowyourendo .com/bookresources, I have included some of my favorite cookbooks, websites, and cooking classes to help you even more.

3. As we learned in Chapter 2, many people with endo also suffer from digestive issues and gut dysbiosis. If you notice that you feel bloated no matter what you eat (or you're sensitive to a lot of foods), it's important to check in with your doctor or seek out a GI specialist. For example, if you find that you're sensitive to the nightshade family or onions and garlic, it's not that these foods are bad, it's that your body has a hard time processing them. It also doesn't mean that you can never eat them again. You might just need to work on healing your gut. Some people with endo have success trying a low-FODMAP diet to begin this process. Understanding a low-FODMAP diet can be a bit complicated, so I recommend working with a nutritionist or buying a book to help guide you through it. There might also be other factors at play that are causing your gut issues, depending on existing food allergies, gastrointestinal diseases, and/or autoimmune conditions that a doctor will be able to help diagnose for you.

And if you have any specific allergies or another condition that might affect your food choices, continue to put those first. For instance, if you have celiac disease, you know that you need to stay away from gluten 100 percent of the time, or if you are on certain medications that do not permit certain foods, do not eat them.

4. Good foods will not cure your endo, but it might be possible for you to manage your pain and symptoms with food in ways you didn't think were possible. No matter how great you begin to feel with your diet changes, please make sure to continue to get checkups with your doctor.

Okay, head to your Good Foods Promise and recipes!

Good Foods Promise

Please follow the schedule in this section.

Every day this week, I promise to:

• Listen to the cues my body is telling me after I eat. These cues might come twenty-four to forty-eight hours later, but I'll still be listening and tracking how I feel.

• Hydrate my body and mind with lots of water each day.

• Read every food label before purchasing something.

• Not be hard on myself if I'm not perfect and remember the reason I want to do this is to **feel better.**

Monday: Eat at least one whole-food, 100 percent plant-based meal (no animal products) today.

Tuesday: Eat at least one whole-food, 100 percent plant-based meal (no animal products) today.

Wednesday: Eat at least one whole-food, 100 percent plant-based meal (no animal products) today.

Thursday: Eat at least two whole-food, 100 percent plant-based meals (no animal products) today.

Friday: Eat at least two whole-food, 100 percent plant-based meals (no animal products) today.

Saturday: Eat at least two whole-food, 100 percent plant-based meals (no animal products) today.

Sunday: Eat all whole-food, 100 percent plant-based meals (no animal products) today.

RECIPES

BREAKFAST

Sweet Potato Breakfast Bowl

Serves 2 to 4

This breakfast bowl is super filling, and the leftovers are great for lunch or dinner, too. Avocado, hot sauce, and salsa aren't mandatory toppings . . . but I really think they make it even better.

2 medium-large sweet potatoes, cut into 1-inch cubes

1½ teaspoons ground cumin

½ teaspoon chili powder

Olive oil

Salt

2 garlic cloves, diced

1 poblano pepper, chopped

1 cup chopped fresh tomatoes

2 cups chopped kale (I prefer lacinato/dinosaur kale)

1½ cups cooked black beans (drained and rinsed if canned)

Preheat the oven to 450°F and line a rimmed baking sheet with parchment paper.

Toss the sweet potatoes with the cumin, chili powder, a glug of olive oil, and a pinch of salt. Place on the prepared baking sheet.

Roast for 35 to 40 minutes, tossing the sweet potatoes a few times, until fork-tender.

While the sweet potatoes are roasting, heat a glug of olive oil in a large pan or cast-iron skillet over medium heat. When the oil is hot, add the garlic and sauté for about 30 seconds, until fragrant. Add the poblano peppers and tomatoes and cook, stirring occasionally, until the peppers soften, about five minutes. Stir in the kale and beans and cook for another few minutes, until the kale softens.

When the sweet potatoes are finished, add to the pan and stir to incorporate all the veggies together. Spoon into bowls and top with avocado, hot sauce, and/or salsa.

Kitchen note: Add a little cayenne to the spices for an extra kick.

Herby Breakfast Sandwich

Serves 2

I'm a fresh-herb freak, so I've always got a bunch in the fridge. If you don't have any on hand, chop up some celery leaves (the little leaves on the celery you usually throw away—they have a nice kick to them), sprouts, or any other greens you have.

4 pieces sprouted or sourdough bread or 2 English muffins, split (Ezekiel muffins are my favorite for this)

2 tablespoons tahini

1 tablespoon white or chickpea miso paste

2 tablespoons freshly squeezed lemon juice

1 tablespoon water

Salt

1 avocado

Handful of fresh herbs (dill, cilantro, and parsley make a good combo for this), coarsely chopped

Toast the bread.

While toasting, in a small cup or bowl, mix together the tahini, miso, lemon juice, water, and a pinch of salt until smooth. Taste and add more lemon juice or salt if you want it. Spread the tahini-miso sauce on two pieces of toast or the bottom halves of the English muffins. Load them up with avocado and herbs. Top with the other two pieces of toast or English muffin tops, mash them together, and eat!

Ingredient highlight: Tahini is sesame seed paste used in Mediterranean and Middle Eastern cuisine. If you've ever eaten hummus before, you've most likely had tahini (it's a star ingredient). You can usually find tahini in the ethnic foods aisle or near the peanut butter or condiments sections at the grocery store.

Fruity Coconut Oats

Serves 2 to 3

I love making a batch of these oats and eating them all week. Feel free to riff on this recipe by adding a combination of different fruits, spices (cardamom or nutmeg work great here), or vanilla bean to make it different every time.

1 cup diced fruit (like berries, pineapple, or peaches)

1 cup canned full-fat coconut milk

1 cup rolled oats

½ cup almond or oat milk, plus more if needed

1 teaspoon ground cinnamon

1 tablespoon chia seeds

Sea salt

Pure maple syrup or raw honey (optional)

Combine the fruit, coconut milk, oats, milk, cinnamon, chia seeds, and a pinch of salt in a large jar or container with a lid. Taste, and add maple syrup or honey if desired. Seal and refrigerate the mixture overnight. Taste it in the morning and add more milk to reach the preferred consistency.

Yogurt Parfait with Chunky Tahini Granola

Serves 2 to 3

This granola isn't super sweet, so it pairs really well with the fruit and yogurt, making this parfait a little salty, a little sweet, and a little crunchy. You can add a bit of cocoa powder to the oats and nuts before you stir in the wet ingredients, to add a chocolate vibe to your batch.

1 cup raw walnuts or pecans (or a combination of both)

1 cup rolled oats

¼ teaspoon sea salt

¼ cup unsweetened flaked or shredded coconut

¼ cup pure maple syrup

¼ cup tahini

2 teaspoons vanilla extract

2 tablespoons coconut oil, melted

2 cups dairy-free yogurt

2 cups chopped fresh fruit (like berries, peaches, pears, mango, or a combination of a few)

Preheat the oven to 350°F and line a rimmed baking sheet with parchment paper.

In a food processor, pulse the nuts until they are broken up a little (but you still want some chunks). Add the oats and salt and pulse 10 to 15 times to break up the oats a bit (but not too much, so they are still mostly intact).

Transfer the oat mixture to a medium bowl and stir in the coconut pieces, maple syrup, tahini, and vanilla extract until combined. Add the coconut oil and give it another couple of stirs.

Press the mixture onto the prepared baking sheet. Spread into a thin, even layer, making sure there are no gaps where parchment paper shows through. Keeping it together will create the chunky bites.

Bake for 12 to 15 minutes, until the edges are slightly browned. Remove the pan from the oven and let it cool without touching the granola for at least 15 minutes. Then break up the granola with your hands into big chunks.

Scoop a serving of yogurt into a bowl. Top with the fruit and granola.

Store extra granola in an airtight container for up to 2 weeks.

Green Smoothie

Serves 1

This is a good starter smoothie if you're new to them. If you're still getting used to the taste of greens, add the minimum amount in the recipe. Next time, add a little more. Eventually, you'll land on a smoothie that is mainly greens with a little fruit. And remember to blend! It's not just a quick whiz in the blender. You need to blend long enough that all the bits and pieces become smooth and creamy. Depending on the power of your blender, this might take a few minutes. Keep going—it will be worth it!

1 to 3 big handfuls of spinach

½ to 1 cup unsweetened dairy-free milk

1 big handful of frozen fruit (like blueberries, pineapple, banana, or strawberries)

1 tablespoon nut butter

ADD-INS

Coconut butter

Hempseeds

Chocolate or vanilla protein powder

Flax meal

Blend the spinach and milk in a blender until nice and smooth. Add the fruit, nut butter, and any add-ins and blend again. Add more milk if needed. Pour into a glass and drink up.

MAINS

Red Lentil Veggie Soup

Serves 4 to 6

I make a batch of this soup nearly every week. It's super easy to make, and I always seem to have the ingredients on hand. You can add more heat by adding the whole jalapeño, and if you don't have spinach, chard or kale will work great here, too.

4 cups + 2 tablespoons veggie broth

1 medium yellow onion or large fennel bulb, chopped

3 garlic cloves, minced

2 carrots, peeled and chopped

2 celery stalks, chopped

1-inch piece of fresh ginger, peeled and minced

1 cup chopped fresh tomatoes

½ jalapeño pepper, seeded and diced

1 teaspoon ground cumin

1 teaspoon turmeric

Salt

1 cup red lentils, rinsed

1 tablespoon tamari

3 cups fresh spinach, chopped

Black pepper

In a medium-large pot, heat 2 tablespoons of the veggie broth over medium heat. When it's hot, add the onion (or fennel) and sauté for 5 to 7 minutes, until soft and translucent. Add the garlic, carrots, celery, ginger, tomatoes, jalapeño, cumin, turmeric, and a pinch of salt and cook for 3 to 5 minutes, until the veggies become soft. Add the remaining 4 cups broth, the lentils, and tamari. Bring the mixture to a boil and then reduce the heat to low.

Cover and simmer the soup for 30 minutes, stirring rapidly every 5 minutes to help break down the lentils. Set a timer if you need to be reminded to stir throughout. Add the spinach and stir until wilted.

Add salt and black pepper to taste and add more veggie broth if you want a more soupy consistency.

Ingredient highlight: Tamari is a gluten-free soy sauce that can be found in the Asian foods section of the grocery store.

Broccoli Coconut Soup

Serves 4 to 6

After a surgery, I ate this soup from Sarah Grossman and Tamara Green's cookbook *The Living Kitchen* for three days straight. It was light but also filling and super nourishing. I felt like it was helping me heal a little bit every time I ate it. Post-surgery, this recipe is a staple in my house, and I'm so grateful Sarah and Tamara allowed me to share it with you here!

1 tablespoon virgin coconut oil

1 large yellow onion, diced

3 garlic cloves, minced

1 large bunch of broccoli, chopped into florets and stalks, peeled

¼ teaspoon sea salt

Pinch of freshly ground black pepper

3 cups veggie broth

1 cup canned full-fat coconut milk

3 cups fresh spinach

TOPPING IDEAS

Lightly toasted cashews or coconut

Sliced green onion

Crunchy Miso Chickpeas (page 165)

Heat the coconut oil in a large pot over medium heat. Add the onion to the pot and sauté for 5 minutes, or until soft and translucent. Stir in the garlic and sauté for another 30 seconds, or until fragrant.

Add the broccoli florets and peeled stalks to the pot and stir to coat them in the oil, onion, and garlic. Add the salt and pepper. Pour in the broth and coconut milk. Cover the pot, bring to a boil, then reduce the heat to a simmer. Let cook for 20 minutes.

Once the broccoli is tender, add the spinach. It will cook quickly in the hot liquid. Let the soup cool slightly and then carefully pour it into a blender. Blend the soup until creamy. Be careful during this step because the soup will be very hot. Blend on low to start, hold the blender lid down firmly with a towel, and don't overfill it, then incrementally increase the speed. Once blended, season with more salt and pepper to taste.

Top your soup with one (or a few) of the topping ideas for added protein, fat, and flavor.

Store sealed in the fridge for up to 3 to 4 days.

Taco Salad

Serves 2 to 3

This salad is especially great during the summer, when corn and tomatoes are in season. It's also great with some crunched tortillas in the bottom of the bowl and some on top, to really make the taco thing happen. Avocado and hot sauce are great additions, too!

1 cup cooked black beans (drained and rinsed if canned)

1 cup corn kernels (fresh off the cob if you can)

1 cup cherry tomatoes, halved

½ cup cooked quinoa

Handful of cilantro leaves

Salt

Favorite greens (I love romaine and spinach for this salad)

FOR THE DRESSING

1 small jalapeño pepper, seeded and chopped

¼ cup freshly squeezed lime juice

1 tablespoon olive oil

½ teaspoon pure maple syrup

TOPPING IDEAS

Avocado

Tortilla chips

Hot sauce

Salsa

In a medium bowl, combine the black beans, corn, tomatoes, quinoa, cilantro, and a pinch of salt.

Make the dressing: in a blender, whiz together the jalapeño, lime juice, olive oil, and maple syrup until smooth.

Pour as much of the dressing as you wish over the black bean and corn mixture and gently mix until everything is coated. Fill up your bowl (or as many bowls as you're serving) with mixed greens. Add scoops of the black bean and corn mixture on top of the greens. Salt to taste. Add as many toppings as you'd like and serve.

Store any of the extra black bean and corn mixture sealed in the fridge for up to 1 week.

Lemon Caper Arugula Pasta

Serves 4 to 6

When I was recipe testing this dish, I had my neighbor try the first batch and her response was "More capers!" I had her try the second batch and her response was "Perfect . . . but still more capers!" I agreed. They really do add a nice richness to the dish, but I know not everyone loves capers as much as we do. I left the measurement of the capers a little open, so you can decide how caper-y you want this to be.

16 ounces spaghetti noodles (I like brown rice spaghetti noodles)

3 garlic cloves, sliced super thin

Zest of 1 small lemon

Juice of 2 small lemons (you can use the lemon you zested)

3 tablespoons olive oil

⅓ to ½ cup capers, drained

3 to 4 big handfuls of arugula

Salt and freshly cracked black pepper

Vegan parmesan or nutritional yeast (optional)

Bring a large pot of water to a boil over high heat. Add the spaghetti to the boiling water and cook per the package instructions.

While the spaghetti is cooking, prep the other ingredients: slice the garlic cloves and zest and juice the lemons. Make sure to have everything ready to go for when you drain the pasta water.

When the pasta is finished, drain and set aside.

Working quickly, in the same pot as the pasta, heat 1 tablespoon of the olive oil over medium heat. When it's hot, add the garlic. Move the garlic around the pan until it becomes fragrant, about 30 seconds. Add the capers. Stir to incorporate with the garlic and oil for about 1 minute. Reduce the heat to low. Add the pasta back to the pot and add the remaining 2 tablespoons of olive oil, the lemon juice, and lemon zest. Combine everything together. I like using tongs for this step to really get the pasta moving. Make sure to get all the way down to the bottom of the pot to get all the garlic and capers that might be hiding down there.

Gently fold in the arugula, one handful at a time, so it begins to wilt. Turn off the heat and serve with a generous pinch of salt, pepper, and vegan parmesan or nutritional yeast.

Store sealed in the fridge up to 3 days.

Ingredient highlight: Nutritional yeast comes in bright yellow-orange colored flakes that resemble fish food. But don't let their appearance fool you! It adds a nice "cheesy" flavor to dishes and can be used in everything from dairy-free mac 'n' cheese to popcorn. You can find it in the vitamin section or bulk section of some grocery stores (and online, too).

Ginger Broccoli Veggie Bowls

Serves 2 to 3

I love this dish for a quick weeknight dinner after work. It doesn't take long to whip up and is super filling with all the veggies. I usually add some seared tofu on top, but any protein will work here. If you can't find bok choy at your grocery store, you can sub in more greens. And the chili paste is a must!

2 tablespoons rice vinegar, plus more as needed

2 tablespoons tamari or coconut aminos, plus more as needed

1½ teaspoons pure maple syrup, plus more as needed

1½-inch piece of ginger, peeled and minced

2 to 4 tablespoons veggie broth, plus more as needed

2 garlic cloves, chopped

1 medium bunch of broccoli, cut into bite-size pieces (about 3 full cups)

1 small head of bok choy, chopped into bite-size pieces (green tops included)

Big handful of chopped fresh greens (kale, spinach, or chard)

Salt

CHOOSE A BASE

Rice, noodles, or quinoa (½ to ¾ cup for each bowl)

TOPPINGS

Protein and/or chili paste (sambal is my favorite)

In a small cup or bowl, combine the rice vinegar, tamari, maple syrup, and ginger. Set aside.

In a large pan, add a splash of veggie broth over medium heat. Add the garlic and move it around the pan until the garlic becomes fragrant, around 30 seconds. Add the broccoli and a couple more splashes of veggie broth, and cook the broccoli until it's bright green and almost fork-tender (don't let the broccoli get soggy), around 5 minutes. Add a little more veggie broth if the pan starts to dry out. Add the bok choy and greens and cook until the bok choy is softened, the greens are wilted, and the broccoli is fork-tender, around 3-5 minutes.

Pour the ginger sauce over the veggies and bring to a simmer over medium heat. Stir until the veggies are well-coated with sauce. Taste, and add more vinegar, tamari, or maple syrup if needed. Salt to taste.

Use the veggies to top the rice, noodles, or quinoa base. Add protein and some sambal chili paste and dig in.

Mediterranean Bowl

Serves 3 to 4

There's a Mediterranean restaurant not too far from my house that lets you build your own "Med Bowl" with a bunch of dips, sauces, and veggies. After paying a lot of money every time I went there, I realized how easily I could make these bowls at home. The base of this bowl is herby rice, but you could easily sub with cauliflower rice or quinoa if you'd prefer. An inspiration bowl to get you started: hummus, tomatoes, cucumbers, parsley, olives, and a drizzle of tahini and lemon juice.

HERBY RICE BASE

1 cup white basmati rice, rinsed

1¾ cups veggie broth

1 teaspoon olive oil

Sea salt

¾ cup chopped fresh herbs (dill, parsley, and mint are a good combination for this dish)

¼ cup freshly squeezed lemon juice, or more if needed

TOPPING IDEAS

Hummus

Baba ghanoush

Chopped tomatoes + cucumbers

Pepperoncinis

Roasted sweet potatoes

Tahini + freshly squeezed lemon juice

Crunchy Miso Chickpeas (page 165)

Roasted carrots

Red bell pepper slices

Kalamata olives

Lentils

Sauteed greens

Chopped parsley

Hot sauce

For the rice base: Combine the rice, broth, olive oil, and a pinch of salt in a medium saucepan. Let the mixture soak for 20 minutes. Bring the rice to a boil over high heat, reduce the heat to low, and simmer, covered, for 12 to 15 minutes, until the rice is cooked through and no water remains. Turn off the heat and keep it covered for 5 minutes.

Stir the herbs and lemon juice into the rice until everything is well combined. Make sure to get all the rice from the bottom and the herbs mixed together. Taste, and add more salt, herbs, or lemon juice if needed.

Scoop the rice into bowls and top with a combination of toppers (the more plants, the better!).

BLT Salad

Serves 2 to 4

Does this coconut bacon taste just like bacon? No. But when you combine it with the romaine, tomatoes, and creamy herb dressing . . . you definitely get hints of a classic BLT sandwich! And if you're actually craving a sandwich, load up all these salad ingredients between two pieces of sourdough or sprouted bread to get even closer to the real thing.

COCONUT BACON

1 tablespoon tamari

2 teaspoons pure maple syrup

Pinch of smoked paprika

1 cup unsweetened coconut flakes (not shreds—you want the big, chunky flakes)

THE REST

Romaine or Little Gem lettuce, chopped

Tomatoes, chopped

Avocado, chopped

Radishes, chopped

Any other veggies or herbs you love

1 to 4 tablespoons Creamy Herb Dressing (page 167), depending on how many people you are serving

Black pepper

Preheat the oven to 350°F and line a rimmed baking sheet with parchment paper.

In a medium bowl, whisk together the tamari, maple syrup, and paprika. Add the coconut flakes and stir to coat the flakes with the mixture (using your hands can really help in this step).

Spread the coated coconut on the prepared baking sheet and bake for 8 to 10 minutes, until it's a toasty brown. About 5 minutes in, toss the coconut around, and then make sure to check on it often so it doesn't burn. Let cool for at least 15 minutes.

Load up the salad bowls with the romaine, tomatoes, avocado, radishes, and any other veggies you love. Add some coconut bacon and drizzle on some dressing. Top with any other fresh herbs you want and a little cracked pepper.

Store extra bacon sealed in the fridge up to 1 week.

Kitchen note: You can add a splash of liquid smoke to make the coconut bacon smokier!

Creamy Roasted Broccoli + Swiss Chard Lasagna

Serves 6 to 8

The most popular recipe from my cookbook, *One Part Plant*, is my Creamy Mushroom Lasagna. I know if something's not broken, don't fix it . . . but I really wanted to riff on it and create a new version of it here. And I actually might like this version better! I've subbed the mushrooms and spinach from the original recipe with two of my other favorite veggies, broccoli and chard. If you can't find chard, you can easily replace it with spinach (just make sure to up the quantity of spinach to 4 to 5 cups if you do). And I love using no-boil lentil or brown rice lasagna noodles to help this dish come together even faster!

¾ cup raw cashews

3 cups bite-size pieces of broccoli

Olive oil

Salt

1 cup veggie broth, plus more if needed

3 garlic cloves, minced

3 cups chard, ribs and stems removed, cut into thin ribbons

1 tablespoon tamari

10 ounces lasagna noodles

4 cups marinara sauce, store-bought (32-ounce jar) or homemade

Nutritional yeast or vegan parmesan cheese (optional)

Preheat the oven to 425°F and line a baking sheet with parchment paper.

In a small bowl or cup, cover the cashews with boiling water and set aside for 15 minutes while you prep the broccoli and greens.

Toss the broccoli with a glug of olive oil and a pinch of salt. Spread the broccoli on the prepared baking sheet and roast for about 15 minutes, tossing halfway through, until tender and a little crispy on the edges.

Drain the cashews and combine with 1 cup veggie broth in a high-speed blender and blend until the mixture is completely smooth and there are no more cashew bits. This might take up to 5 minutes, depending on the speed and power of your blender.

In a large pan or skillet, heat a glug of olive oil or veggie broth over medium heat. When the pan is hot, add the garlic and cook for about 30 seconds, until fragrant. Add the chard and cook until it wilts and softens. If the pan starts to get dry or the garlic burns, add a splash of water. After the broccoli is finished, transfer the broccoli to the pan with the chard.

Pour the cashew sauce and tamari into the pan with the chard and broccoli. Reduce the heat to medium-low and simmer for 2 minutes to let the sauce thicken, stirring frequently.

Prepare the lasagna noodles according to the package instructions. If they are no-boil, you are ready to go!

Spread a third of the marinara sauce on the bottom of an 9 x 13-inch baking dish. Add a layer of noodles. Cover the noodles with half of the broccoli mixture. Add a layer of noodles. Use another third of the marinara to cover these noodles. Add the remaining broccoli mixture. Add the last layer of noodles and cover it with the remaining marinara sauce.

Cover the lasagna with aluminum foil and bake for 30 minutes. Remove the foil, add a sprinkle of nutritional yeast over the top if you'd like, and bake for another 12 to 15 minutes. Let the lasagna rest for 5 minutes before serving.

Store sealed in the fridge up to 3 days.

DIPS + DRESSINGS + SIDES + THINGS

Crunchy Miso Chickpeas

Makes 1½ cups

I love having a batch of these around to throw in salads, as a garnish for soup, or for a crunchy snack. This is a good base recipe, but after they come out of the oven, toss them with any seasonings or spices you love in order to add a little heat or to create different flavors.

One 15-ounce can chickpeas, drained and rinsed

2 tablespoons olive oil

1 tablespoon white or chickpea miso paste

2 tablespoons freshly squeezed lemon juice

Salt

Preheat the oven to 375°F and line a rimmed baking sheet with parchment paper.

Drain and rinse the chickpeas. Shake off the water. Wrap the chickpeas in a clean dish towel and gently press and rock them back and forth. This will dry them and also take off some of the skins (which will help crisp them up).

Whisk the olive oil, miso, lemon juice, and a pinch of salt together in a large bowl. When everything is combined and smooth, add the chickpeas and toss them in the mixture until coated.

Spread the chickpeas on the baking sheet and roast for about 45 minutes, tossing halfway through, until browned and crispy (watch to make sure they don't burn). Remove them from the oven and add salt or preferred seasonings to taste.

Store on the counter in a glass jar with a paper towel or clean dish towel laid over the top for up to a few days. You can also store in the fridge for up to 1 week, but the counter method seems to help maintain the crispiness best!

Ingredient highlight: *Miso paste is a traditional Japanese ingredient made of fermented soybeans (you can also find chickpea or rice versions). It adds a really nice punch to dressings, soups, and sauces.*

Creamy Herb Dressing

Makes 1½ cups

A simple dressing to use on salads throughout the week, a spread for sandwiches or wraps, or a dip for veggies. I left the herb measurements a little loose to suit your taste buds!

¾ cup cashews

1 cup full-fat canned coconut milk

1 tablespoon apple cider vinegar

½ teaspoon garlic powder

½ teaspoon onion powder

1 tablespoon olive oil

Juice of 1 small lemon, plus more as needed

Salt

1 to 2 tablespoons chopped fresh dill

1 to 2 tablespoons chopped fresh parsley

1 to 2 tablespoons of any other herbs you have on hand, such as basil, oregano, or mint (optional)

Freshly ground black pepper

In a small bowl or cup, cover the cashews with boiling water and set aside for 15 minutes.

In another small bowl, combine the coconut milk and apple cider vinegar and set aside for 10 minutes.

Drain the cashews and place in a blender, along with the coconut milk and apple cider vinegar, garlic powder, onion powder, olive oil, lemon juice, and a pinch of salt. Whiz it together until nice and smooth and all of the cashew bits are broken up. This might take up to 5 minutes, depending on the speed of your blender.

Add the herbs and pulse a couple of times. You want to blend them in but still be able to see them.

Add salt and pepper to taste, and any more lemon juice or herbs, if desired.

Store sealed in the fridge for up to 1 week.

Spinach Basil Pesto

Makes ½ cup

The added spinach makes this pesto a great way to get more greens in your day. Use it as a spread for sandwiches and wraps or as a dip for veggies or crackers. You can also toss this pesto with roasted veggies or pasta.

1 cup fresh spinach

2 cups fresh basil

½ cup walnuts

¼ cup olive oil, plus more if needed

1 garlic clove, smashed

Juice of 1 small lemon, plus more if needed

Salt

Whiz the spinach, basil, walnuts, olive oil, garlic, and lemon juice in a food processor or blender until smooth.

Add a pinch of salt to taste and add more lemon juice or olive oil if desired.

Store sealed in the fridge for up to 1 week.

Ginger Cabbage Slaw

Serves 4 to 8 (depending how you use it)

This slaw can be used in so many different ways—layer it on veggie burgers, use it as a topping for baked sweet potatoes, or just throw it on top of some greens to make a quick salad. Feel free to add any extra veggies you have floating around your veggie drawer—radishes, celery, and cucumbers are great additions.

½ small red cabbage, sliced super thin

1 large carrot, shredded

1 red bell pepper, seeded and diced

1 tablespoon miso paste

1 tablespoon olive oil

2 teaspoons fresh grated ginger

2 teaspoons pure maple syrup

Juice of 1 to 2 lemons

Salt

In a medium bowl, combine the cabbage, carrot, and bell pepper. In a small bowl, mix the miso paste, olive oil, ginger, maple syrup, juice of 1 lemon, and a pinch of salt until smooth (miso paste can be a little hard to get smooth, so you can whiz it in the blender if needed). Pour the dressing over the cabbage mix and use your hands to work it into the cabbage. Taste, and add more lemon juice or salt if you like. Depending on how big your lemons are, you might need to use the juice of 2 lemons to balance out the miso. Cover and let sit in the fridge for 15 minutes before serving.

Store sealed in the fridge for up to 1 week.

Coconut Greens

Serves 4

When I moved down south, I had coconut collard greens for the first time and fell in love. I love eating these greens on a bed of rice or as an easy side. I used kale here instead of collard greens because, depending on the season, collards can be hard to find. P.S. If you want them even spicier, try adding some diced fresh chilies.

1 teaspoon olive oil, coconut oil, or a splash of veggie broth

1 medium shallot or small onion, diced

3 garlic cloves, chopped

1-inch piece of ginger, peeled and minced

Salt

Red pepper flakes

2 bunches of kale (I prefer lacinato/dinosaur for this dish)

1 cup canned full-fat coconut milk

1 tablespoon apple cider vinegar, plus more if needed

In a large pan over medium heat, heat the olive oil. When the pan is hot, add the shallot and cook for 5 minutes, or until soft and translucent. Add the garlic and ginger and cook for another few minutes, until they become fragrant. If using veggie broth, you might need to add another splash here. Add a pinch of salt and a pinch of red pepper flakes.

Add the kale to the pan. It will seem like a lot of kale, but it will wilt and cook down as you go.

Toss the kale around the pan and coat it well with the shallot, garlic, and ginger mixture. Cook for a few minutes, until the kale has turned bright green and wilted. Stir in the coconut milk and let simmer for 5 minutes. Give it a couple of stirs as it cooks.

Add the apple cider vinegar. Heat for another minute or so. Taste and add more vinegar, salt, or red pepper flakes to your liking.

Botanica's Seared Japanese Sweet Potatoes with Salsa Verde

Serves 4 to 6

This recipe comes from my favorite restaurant in L.A., Botanica. I had it once and have never stopped thinking about it! So, I asked my friends at Botanica if I could share the recipe here with you . . . and here we are. These pair really well with a giant salad or veggie burger—and the extra sauce is good on just about anything. Emily Fiffer, co-owner of Botanica, says you can sub the cilantro or parsley with dill, basil, or mint, and that grilling the potatoes makes them even better. And if you aren't able to find Japanese sweet potatoes, Jewel or Garnet can work here, too.

1 medium shallot, minced

1 tablespoon sherry vinegar

1 large garlic clove, minced

1 bunch fresh parsley, finely chopped (you can use stems, too)

1 bunch fresh cilantro, finely chopped (you can use stems, too)

2 tablespoons capers, drained and coarsely chopped

Zest and juice of 1 lemon (zest will be used as garnish)

¾ to 1 cup good olive oil, plus more if needed

Sea salt and freshly ground black pepper

4 medium Japanese sweet potatoes (red-purple skin and pale flesh)

Place the shallots and sherry vinegar in a medium-large jar, stir, and set aside to soak for 15 minutes. Drain the vinegar and reserve (in case you want to add it back in at the end), then add the garlic, parsley, cilantro, capers, lemon juice, and ¾ cup olive oil to the jar and stir well. Add a nice pinch of salt and a couple of grinds of pepper. Stir again and taste. You're looking for a balance of acid and herby freshness. If it tastes too harsh, add a few more splashes of olive oil. If you want it punchier, add a bit of the vinegar back in. Add more olive oil if needed to reach the correct consistency. You want to cover the herbs, not drown them, to create a spoonable sauce.

Bring a pot of heavily salted water to a boil. Gently drop in the potatoes. Reduce the heat and simmer until you can pierce the potatoes with a knife but not to the point where they're falling apart or the skin is coming off. This usually takes 15 to 20 minutes but varies depending on the size of the potatoes.

Remove the potatoes, rinse them in cold water, let them cool, and then halve them lengthwise.

Heat a couple of glugs of olive oil in a cast-iron pan or skillet over medium-high heat. Place the potatoes cut-side down in the pan and sear until nice and caramelized, about 5 minutes.

Stir the salsa verde so you get bits of every component, then spoon it generously over the potatoes. Season with salt, zest the lemon over the top, and serve.

Store extra salsa verde covered in the fridge for up to 3 days.

DESSERTS

Oatmeal Chocolate Chunk Cookies

Makes 15 cookies

One of the first things I did when I decided to eat more whole foods was figure out how to make cookies I could still eat without hurting my stomach. These are those! I use chocolate chips instead of the traditional raisins found in oatmeal cookies, but feel free to sub in raisins if that's more your thing.

1 tablespoon flax meal

3 tablespoons water

1 cup almond flour

1½ cups rolled oats

1 teaspoon ground cinnamon

½ teaspoon sea salt

1 teaspoon baking soda

½ cup pure maple syrup

2 teaspoons vanilla extract

⅓ cup coconut oil, melted

½ cup dairy-free chocolate chunks or dark chocolate

Preheat the oven to 375°F and line a baking sheet with parchment paper.

Make a flax egg: Mix the flax meal and water in a small bowl or glass and set aside for at least 10 minutes.

Whisk together the almond flour, oats, cinnamon, salt, and baking soda in a medium bowl. Combine the maple syrup, vanilla extract, and flax egg in a large bowl. Pour the dry mix into the bowl of liquids a little at a time, stirring as you go. When everything is combined, pour in the coconut oil and chocolate chunks and give the mixture a few more stirs.

Use a heaping tablespoon to drop the dough onto the prepared baking sheet. Bake the cookies for 10 minutes, then check on them. They should feel a little soft, almost undercooked, but a little brown on the edges. If they're not there yet, you can bake them for a minute or two longer, but don't overbake them.

Let them cool for at least 15 minutes before removing them from the pan. They will harden a bit as they cool.

Store them in an airtight container (I like to keep them in the fridge) for up to 1 week.

Roasted Grape Sundaes

Serves 4 to 6

The warm grapes with the ice cream alone is pretty perfect, but I love adding a little crunch to this dessert with Chunky Tahini Granola (see page 146), dark chocolate chips, or salted nuts. If grapes aren't your thing, try roasting strawberries, peaches, or apples. All taste great when roasted and served warm over ice cream.

2 large bunches of seedless grapes, removed from the stem (I like using purple or red for the color of the juice)

Olive or coconut oil

Sea salt

Dairy-free ice cream

TOPPING IDEAS

Chunky Tahini Granola (see page 146)

Dark chocolate chips

Salted nuts and seeds

Coconut flakes

Preheat the oven to 400°F and line a rimmed baking sheet with parchment paper.

Drizzle the grapes with a little olive oil, sprinkle on a pinch of salt, and roast for 20 to 30 minutes, until the grapes begin to blister and pop.

Let cool for about 5 minutes and spoon the warm grapes (and some of the juice left in the pan) over ice cream. Add desired toppings and serve! If you have any leftover grapes, store them covered in the fridge for up to 3 days. They are also great on top of yogurt, pancakes, or waffles.

Date Caramel Balls

Makes 18

These are my go-to for an after-dinner dessert when I'm entertaining friends or family. They make for a small, sweet bite, and everyone is always shocked that the inside is just dates and a little sea salt!

2 cups Medjool dates, pits removed

¼ to ½ teaspoon sea salt

1 cup dairy-free dark chocolate chips

½ cup white or brown rice crisps

Line a large plate or baking sheet (just make sure to use one that will fit into the freezer) with parchment paper.

In a food processor, process the dates and ¼ teaspoon of the salt until the dates become a smooth and thick caramel-type paste. You may need to stop and scrape down the sides to make sure you get all the date pieces combined. When smooth, taste the date caramel and see if you want to add more salt. If you do, process again to combine.

Roll the date caramel into heaping teaspoon–size balls. Place on the prepared plate and freeze for 30 minutes.

Melt the chocolate using a double boiler. If you don't have a double boiler, create your own by bringing a few inches of water to a simmer over medium heat in a small saucepan. Place a glass or metal bowl that fits snugly on top of the saucepan, making sure the bowl doesn't touch the water or have steam coming up the sides. And also make sure the bowl and spoon you'll use to stir are completely dry.

Add the chocolate, stirring occasionally, until completely melted and smooth. Remove from the heat.

Drop the caramel balls into the chocolate and roll them around until completely covered. Scoop them out with a fork and shake them a little so that the extra chocolate falls through the tines. Transfer back to the plate and sprinkle rice crisps over the top.

Freeze for another 30 minutes to 1 hour, until the chocolate has hardened.

Store in the freezer for up to 2 weeks.

A Cup of Something Sweet

Serves 1

There are days (and nights) when I'm craving a sweet treat but don't want to bake something or commit to full-on dessert, and this is what I make. It's not exactly cookie dough and you couldn't really bake it, either. So it's truly just a "cup of something," and it always hits the spot.

Big spoonful of nut butter

Spoonful of pure maple syrup

Drop or two of vanilla extract

Pinch of gluten-free flour (brown rice, oat flour, etc.) or oats

Tiniest pinch of salt

Mix-ins options: dairy-free chocolate chips, cacao nibs, raisins, blueberries

Mix the nut butter, maple syrup, and vanilla extract together. Add the pinch of flour and salt and mix all together. Gently fold in the desired mix-ins. Eat it!

Week Four: Movement

One of the things that used to frustrate me most when I was debil-itated in bed with pain was going online looking for answers and reading all the articles, medical websites, and blogs telling me that ex-ercise could make my cramps and endometriosis pain go away. *Really?* If I wasn't able to pick myself up off the couch to take a shower, how on earth was I going to muster up the strength to get on a treadmill? I felt like all the doctors and wellness experts advising this had never had a bad cramp a day in their lives. But after seeing this advice over and over again, that frustration turned into a weird feeling of shame that maybe I wasn't doing enough to manage my pain. If exercise was helping so many people with period pain, was I just a wimp who couldn't manage to pull herself out of bed? Were my symptoms really that bad, or were they just in my head?

That shame and confusion reached an all-time high one winter when I asked for workout clothes for Christmas. They weren't even something I really wanted, but I was determined to exercise to help my pain (just like all the websites told me to). I thought if I ditched my ratty sweats and T-shirts for really expensive leggings, I'd magically have more energy and be excited to hit the gym. I pictured myself with my new gear looking like I just landed in a Nike commercial—with pretty beads of sweat dripping down my body as I boxed, jumped rope, and gracefully whipped those battle rope things up and down on the floor. But on Christmas morning when I opened those new clothes, something very different happened. I faked a giant smile, thanked my dad and my stepmom, Deb, and slipped out of the room to cry. I remember like it was yesterday, sitting in my little sister's very pink childhood bedroom, bawling my eyes out on her bed. Dad and Deb were confused (*Isn't that what she asked for? Does she not like the color of the leggings?*). My sister thought I was overreacting. And I felt like an ungrateful brat crying over Christmas presents. Keep in mind, I was a grown woman when this happened (I wasn't five years old). What my family didn't understand, and what I was too embarrassed to share, was that the fantasy of whipping around those battle ropes wasn't going to happen. Those new clothes didn't make my pain go away, and they didn't magically give me more energy to hit the gym, either. They just reminded me of what I couldn't do.

It was such a scene that Deb put a ban on any of my siblings asking for workout clothes again for Christmas. This ban is still in place, by the way. I can sort of laugh about it now, but at the time it felt like a punch in the gut. I was embarrassed and ashamed that my endo wasn't just affecting me. It was impacting my family, all the way down to their Christmas lists.

Fast-forward to today, and exercise is a giant part of my endo management system. I almost feel the need to apologize to all those articles, blogs, and websites for cursing them all those years. Because they were right—exercise really can help with pain management. But it would be a half-apology, because I feel like they only told me half of the story. It's not as simple as "exercise helps cramps." It's much more than that. Just like food, not all exercise is created equal. You need to find what works for you, and that might change each day. They also forgot to mention that exercise impacts way more than just our physical bodies. It can be a game changer for our endo mental health, too.

Before we go any further, I'm going to stop using the word "exercise" and call it "movement." The word "exercise" makes me think of being exhausted, it sounds like something I can't always do, and like something only those buff bros at the gym can do. But "movement" makes me think of lightness, something I can manage in different ways on different days, and a gentle energy. That's not to say that *your* movement needs to be light and gentle or that being a buff bro is a bad thing. Some friendos thrive doing intense workouts and enjoy more extreme ways of moving their bodies, like competitive weightlifting and boxing. If that's something that makes your body feel good, keep going! The point is, by reframing the word "exercise," we're able to open up our minds about the ways in which we practice it and what's possible for our bodies.

Why Is Movement So Important for People with Endo?

Our bodies: We've all heard about the benefits of movement—from weight loss and heart health to better sleep and clearer skin, but it's rare that we get a full picture as to why movement is so critical for people with endometriosis. Heba Shaheed, a physical therapist we heard from earlier in the book who specializes in working with people who have endometriosis (and has endo herself), sums it up like this: "Because people with endometriosis often spend a lot of time in pain, often curled up in bed, the muscles and connective tissue in the pelvis, abdomen, back, and hips can become tight and sore as well. It's important to keep the body moving to allow the muscles and connective tissue to lengthen, and to allow the nerves to slide and glide freely within the tissues."[1]

Read that last sentence again. Let it really sink in.

Because this week, we're not focusing on movement as a way to lose weight or get a tighter booty. We're using movement to get your muscles and connective tissue moving and to create more calm in your body. We're using movement as a fundamental tool to try to manage your endometriosis better. This mindset shift is important. Just as you are learning how to change your mindset about food, you're going to learn to change your mindset about movement. So, let's dive a little deeper into the reasons movement is so important.

What is your endo motto?

Do what you can during the flare-ups and make the most of your flare-downs.

—Kellie

So much of it comes down to fascia. Heba explains that all bodies have fascia, which is a band of elastic, connective tissue present throughout our bodies. It's the tissue that links everything together. Our fascia covers all of our organs and muscles, and it gives support to our pelvis and spine. The abdominal and pelvic area has a lot of fascia, which is the central core of our bodies (and the part of the body that can cause those with endo some of the most significant pain). Heba says to think about our fascia being similar to the plastic wrap we use in our kitchen. In most bodies, the fascia/plastic wrap is smooth. But in people with endo, that fascia gets scrunched up from inflammation, from endometriosis lesions, or simply from muscle tightness due to clenching your abdomen month after month curled up in bed. If the central core of your body (your abdomen and pelvis) is scrunched up, the rest of your body will follow. Heba explains (and this might be the most important sentence of this chapter), "Neglecting movement can put you at risk of increased pain."

How Do We Begin to Smooth Out Our Fascia?

Abdominal massage is a great way to begin to smooth out your fascia in the abdominal area (see the end of this chapter for a guide on how to do this). Heba says that abdominal massage is "nonnegotiable" when she's working with a patient. This massage technique can help give you more range of movement, help your digestive system, and help your pelvic floor relax. It's important to note that, because so many people with endo have experienced trauma in that area of their body, they might not feel comfortable touching themselves there. If you're not comfortable touching yourself yet, Heba suggests to start by simply putting your hands over that area with a light touch. More on this when she guides you through abdominal massage at the end of this chapter.

Does That Mean We Should Just Focus on Our Abdomen and Pelvic Area to Release Pain and Smooth Our Fascia?

Not exactly. With endo, we tend to think that everything is focused in our pelvic area, but Heba says, "If you have a chronic disease like endometriosis, it's not just the pelvis anymore. You have to look up and down the body." For example, using massage balls can address the pelvic area and help smooth out fascia in different parts of your body, too. Did you know that the nerves in your feet are actually connected to the nerves in your pelvic floor? Pretty wild, right? So, rolling a Franklin ball (or any massage ball) under your foot can assist in fascia release. Foam rolling is another great way to work your fascia. Heba says to think of a foam roller as a giant rolling pin that is able to target a lot of muscle groups at the same time and iron out the fascia. A lot of people with chronic pelvic pain also have tightness in their calf and tibial muscles, and you can use the foam roller to help release these muscles, which will in turn cause "a synergistic release of the pelvic floor as well, because they're connected."

Foam rolling and using massage balls can be incredibly relaxing and a great way to start smoothing out your fascia, but depending on how sensitive your body is, it can be painful at first. Make sure to find the right density (firm or soft) and style (spiky or smooth) of foam rollers and/or balls that work for you. You can also start slowly and work your way up to addressing different parts of your body. For instance, if your legs are super sore right now, start foam rolling on your shoulders first, and when you feel comfortable, maybe move down to your butt. A lot of this work is building trust with yourself and confidence in using these new tools to move your body. And it might feel awkward at first. I remember I rolled right off that roller and onto my butt the first time I used one. Just keep going, and trust that you'll only get better.

I want to assure you that if you feel like you have a body full of scrunched-up fascia right now, that's okay. That's what this week is all about! We're learning more about what our bodies need and why. Later in this chapter, you'll find examples of gentle movements to help smooth it back out.

Our Minds: Even if you know that neglecting movement might put you at risk for increased pain, that doesn't mean you're going to do it. Even if I tell you all about the studies that show that movement can reduce inflammation in the brain (which helps protect against anxiety, depression, and feelings of loneliness),[2] and that people who move their bodies reported greater satisfaction with their lives, it doesn't mean you're going to go grab your shoes and go for a run.[3] Understanding the why is only half the battle. Actually moving your body is a whole other story.

We can come up with a dozen reasons each day not to move our bodies, with excuses involving work, school, kids, and commitments to our friends and family. There are also lots of us who just feel too sad and/or in too much pain to pick ourselves up and move in the first place. Remember the Christmas Workout Outfit Meltdown story from the beginning of the chapter? Yes, my pain contributed to my resistance to move my body, but I was also really depressed because of that pain. And depression can give us zero motivation to move our bodies. This lack of movement can make us even more depressed—yet another vicious cycle that endo can create.

But it's not just feelings of depression that are stopping us from moving our bodies. It's common for people with chronic pain (and specifically people with chronic pelvic pain) to avoid movement for fear of increasing their pain. This behavior is called fear avoidance, meaning that the anticipation of pain can make us want to avoid activity and movement altogether, no matter how much we know it's good for us. Dr. Robert Gatchel, a psychologist who has studied this phenomenon, explains, "Negative catastrophic cognitions lead to avoidance of activities and hypervigilance in monitoring bodily and pain sensations, followed by withdrawal from recreation and family activities, which then can lead to depression, physical disuse, deconditioning, and disability. The formation of these self-imposed barriers to physical activity, in particular, leads to the formation of a negative-feedback loop, which further compounds the cyclical nature of physical decline."[4]

Sound familiar? We talked about catastrophic thinking patterns and pain catastrophizing in Chapter 3. As a refresher, it's when we flood our minds with negative and catastrophic responses to anticipated pain. So, how does this apply when it comes to moving your body? Well, when you have endo, you might already be experiencing pain and/or tight muscles due to lack of movement (again because of your endo). When it comes time to move your body, you get scared. Maybe you start to move your body and then stop halfway through a workout because you anticipate the pain that might follow. You might be scared that moving your body will cause increased pelvic pain or make your muscles hurt even more. Maybe your catastrophic thinking kicks in: *If I work out, then my pain might be worse. It might even rupture a cyst. Which means I won't be able to get out of bed. Which means I will have to miss work. Which means I might be seen as weak or even get fired. Which means I'll be out of a job. Which means I'll have no money.* Once you hop on the negative-thinking train, it's hard to get off. So, you don't move your body. And you don't move your body the next day, and the next. And then your period starts, and you're for sure not moving it then. And then a month goes by without moving your body. And your fear-avoidance behavior continues, which ultimately can increase your pain, create weakness in your body, and make it that much harder to move your body again.

On the flip side, Heba says there's also a "Boom-Bust" personality. This is when you have days that you think, *Oh my gosh, I actually feel really good today, so I am going to do as much as I can!* But then you do so much that you crash, and you can't do anything for a while. When you feel good again, you boom it out and then bust again, boom, and bust. It can be a mental and physical roller coaster.

So how do we avoid our limiting behaviors, break the no-movement or boom/bust cycle, and tap into the power of movement as a management tool?

Pacing

The first step is pacing. Heba explains that pacing is "starting with small achievable goals. We want to change the negative neuro tags from 'this hurts' to 'I can do this much and I feel okay.'" When negative thoughts arise, check in with yourself and be honest about what's possible. There are days when you might feel too fatigued to lift weights, so you make a goal to do a gentle foam rolling routine at home. On the first day of your period, everything might feel like too much, but doing Viparita Karani a.k.a. Legs-Up-the-Wall (which is literally just putting your butt up against the wall and resting your legs straight up on it) is doable. During other parts of the month, you might be able to handle a kickboxing video on YouTube or have a solo dance party in your kitchen while cooking.

Pacing might also include approaching movements you fear in a new way. Last year, I joined a gym with ultra-high-intensity classes, which is something I never thought I would or could do. But after it opened up across the street from my house, I watched the community aspect of it all—so many high fives and cheering "you can do this!"—and I really wanted to join. (I have also secretly always wanted to flip a giant tire.) But after only a few sessions, I quickly learned that those classes were not for my body, no matter how many high fives I was getting. This shouldn't have come as a huge shock to me. I actually knew the research about how high-endurance workouts can spike some people's cortisol and/or create more inflammation in the body. But because I was feeling so healthy and strong, I thought that if I wanted it badly enough, maybe those things wouldn't be true for me. But I was wrong. After my classes, my body felt more inflamed than ever, my fatigue went through the roof, and my body hurt (more than just being sore from a good workout). So, I quit. After I quit, I felt a little embarrassed walking by the gym every day and also a little sad watching all the people still high-fiving one another and reaching their goals.

Walking by that gym one year later, I had an epiphany. Just because my body couldn't do those classes didn't mean I had to quit it altogether. What if I could do it on my terms? I asked one of the owners of the gym if they offered one-on-one sessions that could be tailored to my body's capabilities. I gave him a brief rundown about why I quit, my endo, my fatigue during certain times of the month, and my goals (to get stronger and feel more confident). To my surprise, he responded with a very enthusiastic "YES!" He was really excited for me to come back and really wanted to help me feel stronger, on my terms. Pacing has helped me feel confident in what I'm capable of, instead of feeling like a quitter whose body failed her.

Which endo symptoms do you most despise?

It's the fatigue! For me, it's always been the fatigue.

—Taylor Bryan

Finding What's Best for You

Pacing is a great way to start mindfully moving your body and getting out of the fear/avoidance trap. But in order to this, you also need to find movements your body can (and wants to) do. This sounds so obvious, but the truth is that many of us force ourselves into movements and practices because we see them work for other people. But what works for your friend or for a celebrity you saw online may not work the same for you. And on the flip side, just because someone says a movement isn't good for their endo doesn't mean it won't work for yours.

An Australian survey on endometriosis-management strategies revealed that 15.9 percent of the survey participants said they had increased pelvic pain when practicing yoga and/or Pilates.[5] Does that mean that everyone with endo needs to stop doing Pilates? No way. Jessica Valant, a physical therapist and Pilates teacher (who has endo herself) thrives when she does Pilates. She told me, "I would love to be able to run a marathon. I just can't. And so, I do what I can so that I feel challenged, and I never feel like I'm missing out. And that's what Pilates and yoga both have given me." On the other hand, my sister, Alissa, runs a lot of marathons, does triathlons, and even runs Ragnar races (those long-distance, overnight relays). She loves running, and her body is challenged by it in a good way. Emily Seebohm, an Australian Olympic swimmer, said that when she was first diagnosed with endometriosis it felt like her world got turned upside down. Her first thoughts were: *What do I do with myself? What does this mean for my swimming? What do I do?* She shares that she tried to stay away from reading about what she could and couldn't do—and listened to her body instead. "Reading things online, you start thinking that all you can do is just little tiny things. But I think it's being strong enough to say, 'You know what, I'm going to give my body a shot, and my body can tell me when it's done.'"*

Finding what movement works for you can be a bit of an adventure. You may find that a combination of things works best at certain times of the month. If you've already found what works for you, that's awesome. But if you haven't been moving out of fear—or simply because you just don't love to do it—it might be time to get to the bottom of what's stopping you.

---

* *How comforting is it to hear that even Olympians with endo need a check-in with their bodies?*

Some questions to consider:

- Do you avoid movement because you are afraid you might make your pain worse?
- Are you pushing yourself too hard or not pushing yourself at all?
- Do you find ways not to prioritize movement in your day-to-day life, even though you know it makes you feel better? Why?
- Are you willing to swap out a movement that doesn't make you feel so great and replace it with something new?
- Are you open to trying something that you never thought you could do before?
- Are you able to seek out new ways to practice movement if budget or fear is an issue? For example, if a gym membership isn't in the cards, can you seek out free classes at your community center or try free classes online (movement that you feel more comfortable doing at home)?

I do understand we all have our own set of limitations, from disabilities to what we have access to, but there are *so* many ways to move your body (and so many places to do it) that I'm confident you can find at least a few ways to move. And seeing that this is an adventure to find those ways . . . just for fun (and with an open mind), circle a few things you'd like to try, even if you don't feel like your body is capable of doing them today.

Swimming
Foam rolling
Bike riding
Chair yoga
Rock climbing
Tennis
Tai chi
Tao yin

Golf
Frisbee
Water aerobics
Soccer
Zumba
Dance class
Rebounding
Kundalini yoga

Badminton

Basketball

Kickball

Pilates

Mindful walking (page 107)

Jujitsu

Volleyball

Hiking

Softball

Kickboxing

Karate

Pickleball

Taking the stairs

Boxing

Rowing

Fencing

Racquetball

How'd you do? Did you find some new things you want to try? It's okay if you're still a little fearful of movement or can't imagine yourself ever taking water aerobics (but also, what if it becomes your new favorite thing?). The point of this list is to show you just how many ways there are to move your body. And there are many that you don't have to do by yourself! It's been shown that participating in group movement can decrease your perceived stress and help with your emotional well-being. Not to mention feelings of being less alone and an added sense of accountability.[6]

I struggled a lot with moving my body while writing this book. I was so laser-focused on finishing my first draft that movement felt like it was getting in the way. But I knew if I didn't move, my body would be sore, my periods could be worse, and my depression would slowly begin to creep back in. Accountability is what I needed. So, I asked a friend if she could help me feel more accountable. We lived in different states and couldn't exactly move together, so I would send her a text whenever I moved my body and how. Feeling more accountable and having a buddy to cheer you on can be a game changer. If you're struggling right now, this could be your first step. Tell a friend or family member that you're making a new commitment to moving your body, and that you hope you can share with them when you do. These don't have to be elaborate messages, either. You can simply tell them, "Did it." or "Moved today!"

———

Listening to music can also have a profound impact on your motivation to move, which is something that many of us may have forgotten. These days, we often listen to our favorite podcasts when working out, or watch the little televisions on the gym equipment we use. But neither of these have the same power as music. In Kelly McGonigal's book *The Joy of Movement*, she dedicates an entire chapter to how music can shape our movement. She cites studies and experiments that show how music can "help people transcend their own apparent physical limitations" and that music can reduce "perceived effort, making the work feel easier and more enjoyable." Think about how many athletes you see with headphones on, listening to music as they enter the basketball stadium before a big game or getting amped on the side of the pool before a race. Try it out for yourself the next time you move your body, even if it's just stretching in bed. Turn on some music with encouraging lyrics and/or great beats and see how your mind and body respond.

Ready?

This week, as you begin to move for the first time or continue with your established movement routine, start to envision yourself as "the best" in whatever way you decide to move your body. Start picturing yourself as the Serena Williams of foam rolling, the LeBron James of YouTube Pilates, or the Muhammad Ali of abdominal massage. It might sound silly, but when I'm bouncing on my little trampoline in the middle of my living room, I picture myself as the greatest and most powerful jumper of all time. I become the woman in that Nike commercial I always wanted to be.

Check out your movement promise on page 199, start ironing out that fascia, blast the music, move your body, and envision yourself as the greatest endo-athlete of all time, in whatever way your body can move that day.

Abdominal Massage + Stretches from Heba Shaheed

For beginners, you can put the heel of your hand on your hip bones and middle fingers toward the pelvic bone and apply a gentle pressure upward. After a while of doing this, you might be able to build up to the point where you feel comfortable doing the full massage.

1. Start by lying down on your back.

2. Massage large circles in a clockwise direction in your abdomen—from the hip bones to the ribs to the breastbone and around x 5.

3. Massage smaller circles from the breastbone to 2cm above the belly button x 5.

4. Massage diagonally downward from your right ribs to 2cm above the belly button x 3.

5. Massage diagonally downward from your left ribs to 2cm above the belly button x 3.

6. Repeat steps 3–4 x 3.

7. Massage upward from the pubic bone to 2cm below the belly button x 3.

8. Massage diagonally from the right groin crease to 2cm below the belly button x 3.

9. Massage diagonally from the left groin crease to 2cm below the belly button x 3.

10. Repeat steps 6–8 x 3.

11. Repeat step 1 x 5.

Stretches with Foam Roller

Buttocks Release

1. Sit your buttocks on the foam roller with your knees bent and your feet on the floor.

2. Support yourself by placing your hands on the ground behind you.

3. Cross your right ankle on your left thigh just above your knee.

4. Shift your weight to the right so that you are putting pressure on the right buttock.

5. Roll through the buttock up and down and side to side.

If you find any knots or trigger points, you can hold on each spot for 5 deep breaths.

6. Repeat on the other side.

Front Thigh Release

1. Lie facedown with the foam roller below your hip bones, resting your forearms on the ground.

2. Begin to roll the foam roller down your thighs toward your knees and back up to your hips.

If you find any knots or trigger points, you can hold on each spot for 5 deep breaths.

Back Thigh Release

1. Sit your buttocks on the foam roller with your knees bent and your feet on the floor.

2. Support yourself by placing your hands on the ground behind you.

3. Begin to roll the foam roller down the backs of your thighs toward your knees and back up to your buttocks.

If you find any knots or trigger points, you can hold on each spot for 5 deep breaths.

Back Release

1. Lie back with your feet on the ground and knees bent, with the foam roller under your shoulders and your hands behind your neck.

2. Roll up and down the upper back, mid back, and lower back. You may need to let your bottom rise up in the air to apply pressure to the upper portions of your back as you are rolling.

If you find any knots or trigger points, lean back over the roller into those points and lower the hips; you can hold on each spot for 3 to 5 deep breaths.

Iliotibial Band Release

1. Lie sideways on the foam roller, propping up on your right hand, with the foam roller under your outer right hip.

2. With your right leg straight, bend your left knee and step your left foot forward on the ground in front of your right thigh.

3. Lean into your right hand so that your right arm and your left foot control how much weight is on the roller.

4. Gently roll down the side of your thigh from hip to knee and back up to the hip.

If you find any knots or trigger points, you can hold on each spot for 3 to 5 deep breaths.

5. Repeat on the other side.

Stretches without Foam Roller

Buttocks Stretch

1. Lie on a mat or on your bed with your legs straight.

2. Bend your right knee and bring the knee to your chest, holding the knee gently at your chest with both hands. Feel your hip and groin softening to let go of any pinching feeling in the groin area.

3. Breathe in deeply as you hold this position for a few breaths.

4. Gently press your right knee toward your left shoulder to feel a deeper stretch into the buttock muscles.

5. For a deeper stretch, you can place your right hand on the right knee and your left hand on your right ankle.

6. Hold for 10 deep breaths, focusing on relaxing down your pelvic floor.

7. Lengthen the right leg down and repeat the stretch on the left side.

Groin Stretch

1. Lie on a mat or on your bed with your legs straight.

2. Gently bring both knees in toward your chest, pressing your hands over your knees.

3. Open your hips by pulling your knees away from each other and toward your shoulders as far as you are comfortable.

4. Breathe in deeply as you hold this position for 10 breaths, focusing on relaxing down your pelvic floor.

5. Gently bring your knees back to your chest and lengthen your legs back down to the mat.

Spine Stretch

1. Lie on a mat with your legs straight down.

2. Bring your right knee up to your chest.

3. Using your left hand, pull your right knee across your body toward the left hip as far as you are comfortable.

4. Take your right arm out to the right side, in line with your right shoulder.

5. Hold for 5 deep breaths, focusing on relaxing through the belly and lower back.

6. Repeat the stretch on the other side.

Hip Flexor Stretch

1. Start by kneeling on your knees on a mat (you can have a towel or blanket under your knees).

2. Take a step forward with one foot. Breathe in deeply as you hold this position for a breath.

3. Begin to bring both arms up toward the ceiling. Breathe in deeply as you hold this position for a few breaths.

4. Begin to lunge forward and lift your belly to the ceiling. Hold for 10 deep breaths, focusing on relaxing down your pelvic floor.

5. Relax your arms down, return to kneeling, and repeat the stretch on the other side.

Shell Stretch

1. On a mat, sit on your heels with your knees bent.

2. Curl forward, bringing your forehead to the mat.

3. Reach your arms forward on the mat.

4. If you feel comfortable, you can even take your knees out to the edges of the mat and into a Child's Pose stretch.

5. Breathe in deeply as you hold this position for 10 breaths, focusing on relaxing down your pelvic floor.

Movement Promise

Please follow the schedule below.

Adjust according to your cycle if needed.

Every day this week, I promise to:

• Think about movement as a way to calm my body and smooth out my fascia.

• Practice pacing.

• Find ways to feel more accountable and motivated (text a friend/find new music).

• Have an open mind about exploring new ways to move my body.

Monday: Practice Heba's stretches with or without foam roller.

Tuesday: Walk or do an online/in-person movement class.

Wednesday: Walk or do an online/in-person movement class.

Thursday: Rest.

Friday: Walk or do an online/in-person movement class.

Saturday: Try one new movement practice from the list on pages 191–92.

Sunday: Abdominal massage (however you feel comfortable doing it).

Week Five: Kinder Home + Body

This is our last week together!

After this week, I've got a few more tools for you to discover. But in this last week, we're going to work on creating a kinder home and body.

What do I mean by "kinder"? It means using products that are more gentle, friendly, and safe . . . not only for our home and bodies but for the planet, too. Using kinder products was the last tool I added to my tool kit. Changing my diet, figuring out a movement routine, and having more self-compassion was *a lot* all at once. The idea of transitioning to more natural makeup and cleaning products made my head spin. *What were the best products? Why is natural lip gloss so expensive? How do you know which options are best? But also, why is there such conflicting information about this topic?* It felt completely overwhelming.

But once I hit a groove with my other tools, I was ready to dive in. Surprisingly, this was one of the most fun tools to add to my new kit. It's also the tool that made me feel like I did something really big for myself, with very little effort. I might not be able to take a jog the first day of my period, but I can use my reusable pad. That little bit of care makes me feel proud that I'm doing something for my body that day, even if it's small.

So, as you begin to explore our final tool together, there's no need to panic about having to change everything at once. I'm not going to ask you to throw away all your cleaning supplies, toiletries, or everything in your makeup bag and replace it all with organic, natural products. It would be really expensive to swap everything at once, and you might not be willing to give up your favorite mascara/tampons/face wash just yet. And that's okay.

Just like the other tools, this will most likely be an ongoing process. No matter how quickly or slowly you implement these kinder choices for your body and home, you'll have the information you need to make those conscious choices for *yourself*. Because for far too long, we've been kept in the dark by companies that were not required to disclose their ingredients or share the long-term effects of their products on your health.

You have the right to know about what's going in and on your body.

So, let's get started!

The Disruptors

The first step to creating a kinder body and home is to begin limiting and eliminating products that contain endocrine disruptors. Endocrine disruptors are the chemicals that mimic—and quite literally disrupt—our body's hormones. Dr. Aviva Romm, a women's health expert we heard from a few weeks back, says that this even goes beyond our hormone system: "We actually know that certain environmental chemical exposures, especially estrogenic exposures, change the functioning of our immune system. That reprogramming and that alteration of our immune cells also changes our epigenetics." Which means, "It's changing the way our genes manifest—the shapes of our immune cells." And more studies suggest that endocrine disruptors are involved in the development and severity of endometriosis, in addition to causing health issues such as cancer, infertility, developmental and behavioral problems in children, and asthma.[1]

These endocrine disruptors are everywhere. They can be found in everything from makeup and laundry detergent to menstrual products and even children's toys.

So, what are the biggest endocrine disruptors to watch out for?
- PBDE *found in flame-retardant home products and clothing*
- Parabens *found in makeup, lotions, hair products, and more*
- PFAS *found in nonstick pans, food packaging, stain- and water-resistant products, and more*
- Phthalates *found in plastics and hair-care products, air fresheners, fragrances, makeup, and more*
- Triclosan *found in body wash, antibacterial soaps, and more*
- BPA *found in plastic products, the lining of some canned goods, and more*

After reading this list, you may think you're safe from these disruptors because none of the products you use list these ingredients. But that's the problem. A lot of brands are not disclosing these ingredients to you. For example, the word "fragrance" on the back of your body wash or kitchen cleaner is a catch-all term for over three thousand different chemicals. At the time of writing this, the FDA does not require companies making menstrual products to disclose ingredients on their boxes.* And a 2020 study published in *Environment International* revealed that when seven categories of "feminine hygiene" products (panty liners, pads, tampons, wipes, bactericidal creams, and deodorant sprays and powders) were tested, "24 endocrine-disrupting chemicals, comprising nine phthalates, six parabens, eight bisphenols, and triclocarban," were found in the products.[2] These are products that we put

---

* *In October 2019, New York State passed a bill that will require any period-care products sold in the state to disclose every ingredient on the box. This is a start that will hopefully continue to the national level.*

on, up, and in our vaginas every month—one of the most absorbent and sensitive parts of our body.

Meika Hollender, women's health activist and co-founder of Sustain (a brand that makes natural sex and menstrual-health essentials), explains that there's not a lot of dialogue around these topics the way there is with food ingredients. And because there's not a natural and comfortable conversation happening around periods and the products we use for them, this creates an even bigger stigma around menstruation. So, people don't want to talk about it and are scared to ask questions.

Additionally, there are radically different stances in the debate on how harmful these ingredients are. A quick online search will send you down a rabbit hole with both sides presenting their cases, sometimes making it hard to know what to believe. For example, although there are studies showing parabens (an endocrine disruptor) in products are linked to various health risks, the FDA claims that they do not believe parabens in cosmetics are a danger to our health.[3] Another example is that pads and tampons are made of one of the dirtiest crops in the country, cotton. Because it's so dirty, it's treated with a pesticide called glyphosate, which is believed to be carcinogenic. Yet the EPA says that glyphosate is unlikely to be a carcinogen harmful to humans.[4]

Meika says that "it's hard because there's no pure source of truth, which is true for any health and wellness consumer-product category in general. You have to make your own decision. I think a lot of people have more sensitivity to a tampon that has a synthetic ingredient in it. And some people don't notice it. But other women who have been using these products their whole lives have chronic bacterial vaginosis, and when they switch to nontoxic products, they never experience it again."

The bottom line is that we're just getting started when it comes to learning about the chemicals in our skin care, menstrual, and home products—and the long-term effects of their use. But, with more and more evidence pointing toward the potential detrimental impact these chemicals have on our health, specifically endometriosis—it's worth taking a look at the products you're using and finding kinder swaps for them.

Let's take a look at some!

Menstrual Products

100 Percent Organic Cotton Pads or Tampons

Not too long ago, 100 percent organic cotton pads and tampons came with a much higher price point than their conventional counterparts. They were also more difficult to find. But now, because of public demand, most major stores and pharmacies stock at least one or two 100 percent organic cotton options, and they've become much more affordable. In addition, there are a handful of 100 percent organic cotton tampon and pad brands that have monthly subscription services that deliver right to your door.

If you're not buying 100 percent organic pads or tampons, the product has been sprayed with pesticides and could also include other endocrine disruptors that were discovered in the 2020 study we discussed earlier. It's important to find brands that do disclose their ingredients, so you know exactly what your products contain.

Reusable Pads and Period Underwear

Personally, these two products have changed my entire period world! Reusable pads and period underwear are softer, can be less irritating to the skin, and can bring a sense of freedom, comfort, and peace of mind (no annoying shifting pads, feeling like you're wearing a diaper, or worrying about toxic shock syndrome from an unchanged tampon). And because they are reusable, there is no waste, making them an incredibly sustainable and affordable option, too.

Reusable pads come in a couple of different shapes (some have snaps and others fit into special underwear made for the pads), sizes (liner, maxi, super long), and colorful designs. Leakproof underwear also come in lots of shapes (bikini, night shorts, hip huggers, and even thongs), sizes (there are a lot of size-inclusive brands out there), and colorful designs.

They both work just like a cotton pad. You bleed into the reusable pad or underwear, and it absorbs the blood (some reusable pads can hold up to four tampons' worth of blood). After you're finished wearing them, you quickly rinse them in the sink and throw in the wash, just like the rest of your clothes.

If this sounds gross or you think your periods are way too heavy to try these products, I get it. I was a little squeamish about washing them with my clothes and thought there was no way they'd work with my flow. But I got over it really quickly once I learned how to best use them for my body and because of how much more comfortable I felt on my period. For instance, I am not able to wear *just* period underwear on the first day because of my heavy flow, and I still need a pad. But I can wear my period underwear on the third through fifth days when it's lighter. I also have a special washing bag (that came with my period underwear) that I put my pads and underwear in before I throw them into the wash.

Cups

A menstrual cup is a bell-shaped cup that is inserted into your vagina like a tampon. But instead of absorbing your blood, the cup collects it. Cups can last up to twelve hours, and when it's time to change it, you dump the blood, clean it, and put it back in. This is another great sustainable and affordable option. Because a menstrual cup can last up to a few years, Meika says that can equal about 720 tampons in savings (and 720 tampons and pads not in landfills), which is huge.

If you have issues with tampons irritating or hurting you, cups might not be your thing. But if you're able to wear a tampon comfortably, a cup can be a kinder alternative for your period.

Face + Body + Home Products

Swapping in kinder menstrual products feels like a fairly easy first step, because it's just *one* product. But starting to tackle all the products that we use every day—I'm talking shampoo, conditioner, body scrubs, soaps, lotions, makeup, skin care, deodorants, cleaning sprays, nonstick pots and pans, and even our mattresses—can feel extremely overwhelming.

Like I said earlier, I'm not going to ask you to throw it all away and replace everything this week. And there's also no shame in keeping a few things that you aren't ready to part with. We don't need to be perfect at this, but we can start to be more conscious of our choices.

Here are a few ways to start.

Use the Environmental Working Group's Guides

Just because something says "natural" or "organic" on the label doesn't always mean it's a harmless solution, and it can be really confusing to understand all the ingredients on products (if they are even listed). To help, the Environmental Working Group (EWG) has created trusted comprehensive guides with all the information you need to know about the products you're using and their chemical exposures. You can find guides on everything from cleaning supplies and water to home products (mattresses, paint, and carpets) and more. But my favorite guide they have is called Skin Deep. Skin Deep is an extensive database with over eighty thousand personal care products—including everything from nail polish and toothpaste to sunscreen and perfume. You can type a specific product, brand, or ingredient into their app or website, and EWG gives you a rating on the product's safety on a scale from 1 to 10.

If you want to make changes, these guides are a great way to start. You can use them to plan ahead on the swaps you want to make in your kitchen, bedroom, and bathroom—and discover new, kinder brands and products.

Make a Big Swap

If you're not sure which product to swap first, choose a big one! Dana Bufalino, a board-certified health coach who helps people create healthier skin and homes, explains that when you're starting to make kinder swaps, it's good to start with the largest organ: your skin. She says, "Your cells are drinking whatever you're putting on your body," so the kindest products you can get on the largest surface area, the better. Looking at products that cover the largest areas (body washes, body oils, and lotions) are a great first swap.

After you've made a big swap, go for other important areas like the armpits. Dana says that because our breasts are right next to our armpits, whatever you're putting on them has direct access to your lymph nodes. Start looking into more natural deodorants that don't include endocrine disruptors or aluminum, and use soap or natural oils instead of shaving cream.

In terms of your home, your cookware can be another big swap. If you've been cooking with nonstick pans, consider looking into cast-iron, ceramic, stainless steel, and other kinder cooking options.

Use Your Pantry

There's definitely a stigma around all-natural and low-toxin products being unaffordable and inaccessible to all. And there is some truth to that. There are $100 honey face masks being sold alongside $70 face washes, which might be amazing if they're in the budget (for most they aren't). But you might be surprised at just how many kinder products you can swap into your life using what you already have in your pantry.

Coffee grounds and olive oil can make a great exfoliating mask, and a raw-honey mask can help moisturize your skin. Olive oil and coconut oil can be used all over the body as good moisturizing oils. Vinegar and water can make a great all-purpose cleaner (you can add in a bit of essential oils if you have them on hand, too). And simmering orange peels, cinnamon sticks, and water on the stove makes a great-smelling air freshener.

The point is, you don't have to spend $100 on a honey face mask unless you can/want to. There are hundreds of skin, body, and home-care products you can make straight from your pantry or fridge—ones that require just a handful of ingredients and can be whipped up fast.

What have your gained because of your endo?

Community, tapping into myself, becoming reunited with me.

—Les Henderson

Get to Know Your Skin + Document Changes

I had horrible acne as a teenager. It was so severe that a doctor told me I would most likely not grow out of it and would have adult acne later in life. I was given harsh chemicals to use on my face—along with scrubs, brushes, pads, and different soaps, which only made it worse and created some serious self-esteem issues. I got so frustrated and sad when nothing was working that I decided to throw it all away and defiantly declared that I'd never put anything on my skin again! And that's when my acne went away. That was the first time I started to get to know my skin. Of course those brushes, soaps, and chemicals were making it worse. They were irritating my skin more because it was so sensitive. More isn't more for my skin, and I had to learn that the hard way.

We all have different tolerances for different products. The tampons your friend uses with no problem might cause you a lot of irritation. The natural deodorant that is all the rage may make your armpits break out with a rash (in which case, you might want to look for brands that do not include baking soda and are made for sensitive skin). Get to know your skin and body better by documenting past or present irritations, rashes, discomfort, or headaches. Is there any connection to the products you're using? You might not be able to pinpoint it right now, and this is not to say there's for sure a connection to a product you're using, but continue to document them, take out any questionable products for a week to see if it helps, and just get to know your skin better.

Take a Break

If you load your skin up every day with lotions and oils, body wash, makeup, deodorant, and more, your skin might need a little break. Dana Bufalino, who we heard from earlier in this chapter, suggests having a product-free day once a week, to let your whole body have a chance to really be itself.

It might feel strange at first to only use water in the shower, or to skip your deodorant and your daily face routine. But Dana says doing this even once a week can be balancing and regulating and gives our skin a chance to breathe. This is also a great time to document any changes you see. And guess what? You're going to do this, in this week's promise. Head over and get started!

If you want to find out more about kinder face, body, and home products, I have some of my favorite brands and products at knowyourendo .com/bookresources.

Kinder Home + Body Promise

Please follow the schedule in this section.

Monday: Take inventory and make a list of all the menstrual, skin care, body, and home cleaning products you use. All of them!

Tuesday: On that same list, get to know your skin better by documenting any present or past irritations, rashes, or discomfort you've felt. Are you able to connect them to a product you've used?

Wednesday: Review your list of products you use and choose a few that could be big-swap candidates. Explore EWG's website, kinder beauty brands, and check out some of my favorite resources at knowyourendo .com/bookresources. If you're not able to buy them now, that's okay. The first goal is getting a plan together.

Thursday: Just chill.

Friday: DIY something from your pantry or fridge (a cleaning product, face mask, moisturizer, air freshener, etc.). There are hundreds you can find online, or get inspired by the ones I listed on pages 208–9.

Saturday or Sunday: Choose one day to be your product-free day. No products of any kind. Let your skin breathe!

9

More Tools to Explore

The tools that we're going to explore in this chapter are foundational tools for a lot of people with endo (the same way that good food and movement are for others). I've heard so many stories of how pelvic floor therapy has been life-changing for some, and I know some friendos who can't get through the month without their CBD gummies. I love that these therapies and products can have such a profound impact on managing endo, but depending on where you live, your budget, your body, or your personal belief system, not all of them will be options for you—either right now, or ever.

Heather Guidone, the board-certified patient advocate whom we heard from earlier in this book, explains that "certainly, pelvic floor therapy is very important, but if you can't afford it, it doesn't matter how important it is." But she also says there are some clinical trials and studies for acupuncture and cannabis that you can look into joining, and some pelvic floor therapy and traditional Chinese medicine practices offer sliding scales. And if you do have the budget but live in a city that does not offer these services, some therapists have telehealth options as well.

I do have hope that a lot of these "alternative" therapies, products, and services will become more mainstream and more accessible to all. In the meantime, read through these options, educate yourself, ask friendos about their experiences, and do/choose whatever works for you.

Pelvic Floor Therapy

Like I said, I've heard lots of stories from people with endo having great success using pelvic floor therapy to help manage their symptoms and feel more connected to their bodies. It's not something I had ever tried, and I felt a little strange writing about it without doing it first. So I set up a session with a local pelvic floor therapist, Tracey Manasco, MPT, so I could share some firsthand experience. I know that every practitioner might do things a little differently, but there are some general guidelines of what you can expect at your first appointment.

Before we get into the session, let's talk a little bit more about what pelvic floor therapy is exactly. Pelvic floor physical therapy is practiced by a licensed physical therapist who has specialized training in treating pelvic floor dysfunction. Tracey, who specializes in working with people with endometriosis (and has endo herself), explains that physical therapists are trained to treat the musculoskeletal system (which includes the skeleton, muscles, cartilage, tendons, ligaments, joints, and other connective tissue), and the pelvic floor is a part of this system. "It's a group of muscles that attach primarily from the pubic bone to the tailbone and provide support to the abdominal organs, provide continence of urine and stool, participate in sexual function, and coordinate with other muscles to help with core stability." But there can be problems within this system, including pelvic pain (which can include pain in the bladder, muscles of the pelvic floor, and rectum), painful sex, abdominal pain, and bloating.

Tracey says that pelvic floor therapy can specifically help people with endo manage painful trigger points in the pelvic floor, decrease central sensitization (an overstimulated nervous system), help with tension in the muscles of the pelvic floor, decrease "endo belly," and help manage scar tissue.

In my appointment with Tracey, she first asked me to share my story—any previous surgeries, past or existing pain and symptoms, the lengths of my cycles, and stressors in my life. She also asked me about my diet, sleep, digestion, and any trauma I've experienced (including sexual trauma). Not all pelvic floor therapists ask about diet and lifestyle, though Tracey sought extra training in nutrition because she says that endometriosis is a complex disease that takes a multifactorial approach. She believes that "the pain, fatigue, bloating, digestive issues, anxiety, and depression involve so much more than just the musculoskeletal system."

Next, Tracey had me stand up so she could check out my posture, balance, spinal alignment, patterns in my breathing, and muscle coordination. It was pretty incredible to learn that all of these things can impact our pelvic floor or are altered by a weak one! After that, I lay down on the table for what she called the "fascial and muscular layers assessments." Tracey moved her hands over my abdomen and was looking for any trigger points and adhesions/scar tissue, while also feeling my abdominal fascia. She then started the internal exam. Meaning she used a gloved finger to inspect inside my vagina to assess my pelvic muscle tone, areas of pain, pelvic floor tightness or weakness, and ability to relax.

Tracey explained that not every patient receives an internal exam. Not every patient is ready, mentally and/or physically, for this part of the assessment. If they are not ready, she might first work to help calm their nervous system down, share breathing exercises, and/or do dilator therapy (something we discussed in Chapter 3). Some patients are not able to tolerate a tampon, let alone someone's finger moving around inside of them. Tracey made sure to tell me that we could stop at any time if I was uncomfortable or experienced any pain. She shared that the exam was supposed to assess for pain, not increase it.

After my internal exam, Tracey shared what she found while examining me, and we talked about goals and next steps. These next steps will be different for everyone. But I wanted to share the type of homework she gave me to give you a better understanding of what to expect. She said that because I have bladder issues, she wanted me to start a bladder diary (to record how much water I drink and how often I pee). Tracey also gave me breathing exercises and poses to do at home (Happy Baby, Child's Pose, and Baby Cobra). She also wanted me to do some skin rolling and massage on some of my scars and in the areas that felt tight. The coolest thing about working with Tracey is that she followed up with a video to remind me how to do all these things. This was incredibly helpful, because I did forget about half of the things we talked about as soon as I walked out the door (we covered a lot!).

It's important to note that I felt really comfortable with Tracey, I wasn't experiencing a lot of pain at the time of my visit, and I had worked through a lot of my past trauma before coming in. But if I had felt the slightest bit uneasy with my therapist or was still in a lot of physical or emotional pain, this session could have been a different experience.

For those with endo and/or those who have experienced past sexual trauma, just touching your own body (let alone someone else touching you) can bring up a lot of emotion. This therapy can be a really intimate experience, and I cannot stress enough the importance of finding someone who makes you feel comfortable and is willing to talk you through any emotions that come up. It doesn't matter how great the therapist is or how many amazing online reviews they have—if you don't feel safe and cared for, they're not the therapist for you.

Some other notes:

- Some states require a doctor's referral to see a pelvic floor therapist and others do not. If you are required to have one and are unable to get it from your doctor, you can work with your therapist to refer you to a doctor who will help you.

- While I would typically look for someone in-network, Tracey did not accept insurance. It did feel worth the cost based on the amount of one-on-one time and care that she was able to give me. Some physical therapists are covered by insurance, but before you book, find out how much time they will be able to spend with you and how many other clients they'll be working with at the same time. You might prefer one-on-one care because you know it will be painful or emotional for you—while others are completely fine in a group setting. As always, it comes back to doing what works best for you and what your budget allows.
- Tracey says that the amount of sessions a patient will need really varies, but she typically works with someone for six to eight sessions, sometimes more and sometimes less. And if you are going to make the investment in these sessions, it's important to commit to doing the work at home, too.

We're just skimming the surface of pelvic floor therapy. There's so much more to cover—and if you're interested in learning more, I have more information for some of the best therapists, books, and resources at knowyourendo.com/bookresources.

Herbs + Supplements

If there is one sector of the health and wellness space that gives me pause, it's the supplement industry. There are so many brands making big claims about their dusts, powders, pills, and tinctures that it's hard to know what's what. And it's also really easy to get sucked in by the pretty packaging and promises of life-changing effects by sprinkling something in your tea. A lot of us have cabinets full of these products and are unclear how (and if) they are helping us at all.

During an interview with Giselle Wasfie, a doctor of acupuncture and Chinese medicine and board-certified herbalist, she shared something with me that has become my herbs-and-supplement mantra: *"Herbs work."* Meaning, herbs and supplements can have a powerful positive or negative impact depending on who is taking them. Not all herbs and supplements are created equal, and it's important to be aware of potential side effects, your sensitivity to them, the dose you're taking, and if you're able to combine them with other medications.

If you've never tried any supplements before or feel overwhelmed by the amount you "could" be taking, start by focusing on the ones you know you *need*. If you're able to, getting blood work done once a year to see what vitamins are actually lacking in your system can be really helpful to narrow it down.

For example, deficiencies in B_{12} can lead to cognitive issues, fatigue, weakness, depression, numbness and tingling of the hands and feet, and anemia. And if you are choosing a more plant-based, vegan, or vegetarian lifestyle, B_{12} is a must. Vitamin B_{12} is typically found in animal products or bacteria. So, if you're eating a diet full of meat, dairy, or eggs, you're most likely getting enough B_{12} from the animals that made these foods. The cow that made the steak or hamburger on your plate got its B_{12} from the bacteria that lined its gut or ate a food source (sometimes feces) covered in bacteria. So when you eat that burger, you are essentially getting your shot of B_{12} from the bacteria from the cow that made the steak or burger. Yes, eating more plants can get you almost everything you need in terms of vitamins and nutrients, but nearly all lack B_{12}. You can find certain types of algae, rare mushrooms, and fortified foods (dairy-free milks, nutritional yeast, and cereals) with B_{12}, but these are not typically adequate sources and why you may need supplements.

Vitamin D is another. Deficiencies in vitamin D can lead to depression, fatigue, and muscle pain (symptoms that so many of us with endo face already). A study on vitamin D deficiency in adults showed that the overall rate of deficiency was 41.6 percent, and people with darker skin had rates even higher, with Hispanics at 69.2 percent and Black participants at 82.1 percent.[1] Just like B_{12}, if you're not eating meat or dairy, it's tougher to get your vitamin D from plants, so a supplement could be necessary for you.

These are examples of just two vitamins that you may not be getting from your food or lifestyle, no matter how healthy it is. Getting a blood test can help determine what you may need to add.

In terms of supplements specific to endo, there are so many theories out there about which supplements are best that I could fill this entire chapter with them. I'm reluctant to share a big list because there's not a lot of evidence to support how they specifically work for endo. I also think lists like that can feel overwhelming and expensive, as you tally up the cost of taking a whole slew of supplements.

That said, I do want to share a few supplements and herbs that have been shown to target inflammation, which can help support your endo management plan. I asked women's health physician and herbalist Dr. Aviva Romm, whom we heard from in previous chapters, for her top three supplements for endo management. She suggests N-acetyl cysteine (NAC), curcumin (the extract of turmeric), and ginger root for their anti-inflammatory properties. Dr. Romm shares, "When I approach a patient with endometriosis, it's not like I say, 'Okay. Go home and try NAC for six months.' It's part of a whole picture of diet and lifestyle."

Supplements are just that: they are supplemental to the rest of your tools. You cannot depend on a supplement alone to manage all your endo symptoms. No matter what you decide to take, always do your research, consult your doctor or an herbalist, and remember our herbs-and-supplements mantra: *Herbs Work!*

If you're interested in learning more about herbs and supplements, I have additonal resources at knowyourendo.com/bookresources.

Lymphatic Movement

New studies are showing that the lymphatic system could play a role in the progression of endometriosis. There's not enough evidence to have

*What is your greatest
endo management
tool?*

*Therapy! I feel like a
therapist has helped
me to manage my
anxiety and depression
that runs right
alongside my endo.
Taking control of my
mental health has
been one of the best
tools for managing a
life with chronic
illness.*

—Kendall Rayburn

definitive proof of this yet, but regardless of how much the lymphatic system impacts endo itself, we do know that draining and supporting our lymphatic system is beneficial to our overall health.

So, what is it?

The lymphatic system is a network of blood vessels, tissues, and organs that help cleanse toxins and protect our bodies from infections. Unlike other systems in our body that work on their own, the lymphatic system needs a little help from us. If we're not able to keep the system moving, it can get sluggish and build up toxins, which can lead to fluid retention, chronic pain, and poor immunity (three issues that people with endo can already suffer from).[2]

And how do we keep the system healthy and detoxify?

One of the coolest things about supporting our lymphatic system is that there are pretty simple ways to do it that don't take a ton of time, actually feel really good, require little investment, and are things you may have already started doing in our five weeks together.

- Foam rolling
- Jumping on a rebounder (little trampoline)
- Dry skin brushing before a shower
- Moving your body (walking, yoga, etc.)
- Deep breathing and stress-management practices
- Staying hydrated
- Lymphatic massage

Research a few of these options, find which ones work best for your body, and get your lymphatic system moving!

Traditional Chinese Medicine (TCM)

Traditional Chinese medicine is an ancient Chinese medical system comprised of different healing modalities to help manage and treat illness and disease of the mind and body. For some people with endo, TCM has enabled them to have less painful periods, reduce symptoms and inflammation in the body, improve fertility, and assist in managing the mental health issues from having endo.

To help understand TCM and how it can impact endometriosis pain and symptom management, I called on Jill Blakeway, doctor of acupuncture and Chinese medicine, a clinical herbalist, and one of the most renowned experts and practitioners in the field. Basically, we're in really good hands to better understand this complex management tool.

Jill says that when people think of Chinese medicine, they think of acupuncture, but it's the entire "whole systems Chinese medicine" that helps. It's not just acupuncture. It's a combination of looking for disharmony in the body, dietary advice, lifestyle adjustments, massage, moxibustion (burning of mugwort), cupping, and herbal medicine. And when it comes to endometriosis, Jill explains, "In Chinese medicine, endometriosis isn't just one disorder, because it isn't biomedically either. There are different routes to it. Chinese medicine is all about the way one symptom has meaning in relation to other symptoms."

When looking for a therapist, Jill says to first look for one who is licensed and board certified in both acupuncture and Chinese herbs and has experience in gynecological issues.

You also want to find a therapist whom you feel comfortable with, because it can be a very intimate and personal experience. Jill says she believes that "people heal when they feel safe. And particularly from something as personal and central as endometriosis, it's very central to your life. You can't get away. It's not like you can ignore the pain. It can dominate your life. I think in order to unpack that fully and start to unwind some of the strain around that, you need to feel safe. You're looking for a practitioner who gives you that confidence and safety."

Similar to working with a pelvic floor therapist, in your first TCM visit, your therapist will go deep into your health history and lifestyle and create a plan for your treatment. Jill says it's important for them to set goals with you, and that these goals should be quantifiable—whether that's having less pain, fewer PMS symptoms, or less/no spotting between periods. Having these measurable, realistic, and tangible goals is powerful. She adds, "Be careful of anyone who tells you that they can magically make your endo go away."

In terms of how many treatment sessions you'll need to feel results, Jill says that with endo, it takes a bit of time. She explains, "Even when you make changes to your diet, it takes time for that to work its way through, so it's a bit of a process." She says you should give it two to three months, but you should see improvement after six weeks (again, this is why measurable goals are good).

A lot of TCM practitioners do not accept insurance, but some work on sliding scales. You can also look into community clinics, which can be less expensive.

If you're interested in learning more about TCM, I have links to more information at knowyourendo.com/bookresources.

Cannabis + CBD

I didn't experiment with any drugs in high school or college. I was sort of an alterna-teen who thought it was more rebellious *not* to do what everyone else was doing (a.k.a. drinking and drugs). Years after college, I still had no interest in trying. If I hadn't tried it in my twenties, what was the point in doing it now? But then, at the age of thirty-three and encouraged by a friend who wanted me to experience the amazing benefits of cannabis, I finally smoked weed. And after that night, it became one of my biggest tools to manage my endometriosis pain and symptoms.

Before that night, it had never really occurred to me that cannabis could be used as medicine for endo. But this idea isn't new. As far back as 1564, the German botanist Tabernaemontanus wrote, "Women stooping due to a disease of the uterus were said to stand up straight again after having inhaled the smoke of burning cannabis."[3] And a more current version of this philosophy comes from Maya Elisabeth, one of the most celebrated people in the cannabis industry (and someone much more familiar with having a uterus). She says, "Cannabis is our best ally for menstrual relief and often the most overlooked."

Maya explains there are active components in cannabis called cannabinoids and that our bodies are covered with cannabinoid receptors (including the pelvic area). The cannabinoids work with their receptors like a lock-and-key system. When the lock and key connect, it triggers a reaction in our minds and bodies. When the cannabinoid THC (the compound in cannabis that makes it psychoactive) attaches to a receptor, it creates a reaction that has been shown to help manage pain, inflammation, anxiety, and sleep. CBD is another cannabinoid in the cannabis plant that's also found in hemp plants. However, it does not attach directly to the receptor and is nonpsychoactive (it will not get you high, unless the CBD has THC added to it). Benefits of CBD can include managing inflammation, sleep, and anxiety.*

Maya says that the biggest difference between THC and CBD is, aside from the psychoactive effects, that "one is legal in every state and the other isn't." Cannabis is not yet legal in every state, yet some states

---

* *Cannabis can help some people with anxiety, yet some of its psychoactive effects can increase anxiety in others. Speak to your doctor about using marijuana or CBD.*

What is your greatest endo management tool?

WEED. I use it to have a better and less painful sex life, have an appetite when I am too nauseous to eat, and for daily pain management. It also just makes watching reality TV approximately two thousand times better.

—Lara Parker

allow medicinal use. For example, at the time of this writing, Florida has not decriminalized cannabis, and it's illegal to use it recreationally. But you can legally buy medicinal marijuana from a dispensary with a medical card, whereas hemp-based CBD can be purchased online and in stores, no matter what state you live in.

When buying cannabis or hemp-based CBD, Maya says you need to know your sources. It should be organic, processed clean, and lab tested. It's important to do your research, find brands that have the highest standards when purchasing products, and be wary of CBD brands claiming to cure cancer or stop your endo from growing. That $8 CBD spray sold in the checkout line of your grocery store that promises to get rid of your anxiety is probably not the CBD you're looking for.

Similar to herbs and supplements, your body might process cannabinoids differently than someone else. Depending on the way your body reacts, you may need a higher or lower dose than is recommended. Your experience is your own, and it's important to check in with yourself and not compare your experience with someone else's.

In terms of the best applications of cannabis, they range from bath salts, oils, edibles, and more. Maya also includes suppositories as one of her favorites for pelvic pain, because she says it's essentially applying "a topical to your uterus." It can also work as a great lubricant and help relax your muscles when having sex.*

For some, cannabis and CBD can be a powerful tool for endo man-

---

* The oil in suppositories can break latex, so Maya does not recommend combining the two.

agement. But similar to supplements, they should be used as a supplemental tool (along with your food and lifestyle choices) and not as a quick fix or treatment for your endo.

If you're interested in learning more about cannabis, there is a collection of books, reputable brands, and other resources at knowyour endo.com/bookresources.

Keep Going

It's weird to belong to a club of really strong and amazing people—that none of us really want to be in. We didn't choose to join Club Endo. It somehow chose us. And because we're in this unchosen club together, even if we've never met, I feel a connection to you. Which makes it feel really hard to end this book and say goodbye. I'm not exactly sure how to do it, but here's my best.

Many weeks ago, when you started this book, I told you I wanted so badly for you to get to a place where you could find some endo wins for us to celebrate together. I'm hoping you were able to find a few. Maybe your win was getting out of bed, going to work, or moving your body more. Maybe your win was no longer letting your voice be silent, advocating for yourself, or beginning to better understand your condition. Maybe you discovered new wins you didn't even know you wanted, or you're still trying to find them.

No matter where you are with these wins, *please keep going*.

Keep making yourself a priority.

Keep asking questions.

Keep protecting yourself.

Keep practicing self-compassion.

Keep asking for help.

Keep understanding that not every day will be perfect.

Keep living.

And please, keep remembering that you're not alone.

The aloneness. I think that's why it feels so hard to say goodbye. Because it really wasn't until I wrote this book that I realized just how alone I used to be. And man, was I alone with my endo. I had to tap into a lot of that loneliness to write these pages, and unearthing that brought up old feelings of sadness and rage about how I was treated and how I used to feel. It also brought up new feelings of sadness and rage—about the inequalities in our healthcare system, how hard so many of us have to fight to be heard, and how many of us are hurting. Many nights, I went to bed crying during the writing of this book, and I wasn't always the nicest person to be around.

I should also share that I went to bed some nights crying happy tears because of how hard people are fighting for the endo community with their research and activism. I also bragged a lot about the strong and remarkable people whose stories you heard in this book (which made me cry even more happy tears).

Writing this book was truly a roller coaster of emotions, to say the least, and there were many times I wanted to quit.

But this club of ours is what kept me going.

How could I give up on us? I will never feel alone in my endo ever again, because of us. Because of our stories. And because of how far we've come.

You might feel the sadness and rage some days, but there will be strong and remarkable moments, too. Keep going for all of us. Keep using your tools. Keep believing that you deserve to feel good in your body. I'm going to keep remembering that, too.

All right. I'm ready.

See you later, friend.

Thanks for letting me hang out with you for these past few weeks.

I wish all the hope and health in the world to you.

Love, Jessica

Acknowledgments

I almost didn't want to write this section because I was so afraid I was going to forget someone. If I did, I'm sorry. Tell me and I'll buy you a drink or figure out another way to publicly thank you. OK, here we go . . .

Thank you to:

Amanda Kahle. You didn't mean to change my life, but you did. I'll continue to thank you for the rest of our lives (even though I know it's starting to annoy you).

My agent, Sarah. You are a force. I'm constantly bragging about your willingness to fight for me/this work. Thank you for always responding to my late-night texts . . . even when they have nothing to do with books and everything to do with some show I'm watching. And *Celeste and the entire Park Fine Team.* For everything!

My editor, Lauren. For your patience and kindness. One more shoutout to your patience! Wow. Thanks for changing all my "thats" to "whos" and making this book better. *Megan.* For believing that endometriosis deserved a bigger spotlight. I'll be forever grateful. And to the *entire Avery/PRH team* (design, publicity, copyediting, marketing, warehouse/shipping, and everyone behind the scenes) for working so hard to get this book in people's hands.

The contributors of this book: the doctors, experts, endo advocates, recipe testers/contributors, and friendos who shared their stories. For giving your time and knowledge, and being so willing (and excited) to help with this book. *The Know Your Endo community and everyone who took the Endo Tool Kit Course.* You shaped this book, and I cannot thank you enough. An extra special thanks to *Dr. Goldstein* for helping me with all the ins and outs of endo and all the ins and outs of finding more peace with my body.

My fellow author buds and friends who helped with this book: *Heather Crosby.* Not even sure what to say, because there's so much. I love you, witchy sister. *Serena Wolf and Phoebe Lapine.* For forty-two-messages-deep moral support/goss text chains. *Rachel Holtzman.* For somehow always getting it. How do you do that? *Will Bulsiewicz.* For always checking in on me and believing this book mattered. *Kathryn Budig and Kate Fagan.* For your writing advice and always being up for celebrating wins. *Al Holleb.* For providing my home away from home for work trips and Cyst-gate 2017. *Racine Clark.* For recipe testing, and always asking how my paper was going. And to our H Street/Tez porch hangs that made a strange year less strange. *Huriyali and West Ashley WFM.* For giving me a space to write and never making me feel bad for sitting in that space for soooo long. *Gervais Hagerty.* For showing me what true determination looks like. *Daphne Javitch, Ashlae W., Nina Thompson, Emily Fiffer, Dana Bufalino, Aviva Romm, Elizabeth Stanley, Ruby Warrington, Claire Ragozzino, Katie Horwitch, Katie Dalebout, Ami Murphy, and the Barretts.* For always pushing me (in the best way possible). And *Jessica Duffin, Mozhan Marnò, Kyla Canzater, April Christina, Meg Allan Cole, Lauren Kornegay, Shannon Cohn, and Lara Parker.* My no-bullshit endo sisters who don't quit and inspire me to do the same.

All my parents and sibs: *Mom.* I'm so sorry that no one believed your pain. But I do. And thank you for always believing mine. You taught me true empathy and compassion. *Dadal.* You believed in positive thinking before it was cool (sorry it took me twenty years to finally pull out that

Wayne Dyer book). Thank you for showing me how to teach and be a storyteller. *Debba*. For showing our family how to make every moment special. *Tom and Reen*. For accepting me from day one, even when I was in pain and you didn't know that was why I was being so weird. I wish the world could feel your unconditional love. *Alissa and Kells*. Didn't think we could get any closer . . . thank you for always being so enthusiastic about everything and forever elevating. And *Pickle*, *Abs*, *Christine*, *Yes*, *B*, and *Helen*. I love you all so much.

Sid. For knowing how to say "endometriosis" and throwing me pads. Your special snacks, drawings, and wrestling-match breaks helped me write this book. *My D*. Now the tears have started. It felt weird dedicating an endo book to a dude (so I didn't), but you are one of the biggest reasons I'm breathing and sitting here today. You've been with me through it all but have also given me the space (and without judgment) to be alone and figure it out on my own. I'm going stop right here and go give you a giant hug in the other room. Loooooove.

And thank *you* for reading this book. I really hope we get to meet someday, so I can hear your stories, too.

Notes

Chapter 2: The Ins and Outs of Endo

1. O. Bougie, Ma I. Yap, L. Sikora, T. Flaxman, and S. Singh, "Influence of race/ethnicity on prevalence and presentation of endometriosis: a systematic review and meta-analysis," *BJOG: An International Journal of Obstetrics & Gynaecology* 126, no. 9 (2019): 1104–15.
2. Kelly M. Hoffman, Sophie Trawalter, Jordan R. Axt, and M. Norman Oliver, "Racial bias in pain assessment and treatment recommendations, and false beliefs about biological differences between Blacks and Whites," *Proceedings of the National Academy of Sciences of the United States of America* 113, no. 16 (2016): 4296–301.
3. Paulette Maroun, Michael J. W. Cooper, Geoffrey D. Reid, and Marc J. N. C. Keirse, "Relevance of gastrointestinal symptoms in endometriosis," *The Australian & New Zealand Journal of Obstetrics & Gynaecology* 49, no. 4 (2009): 411–14.

Chapter 3: Life with Endo

1. N. Fritzer, D. Haas, P. Oppelt, St. Renner, D. Hornung, M. Wölfler, U. Ulrichg, G. Fischerlehner, M. Sillem, and G. Hudelist, "More than just bad sex: sexual dysfunction and distress in patients with endometriosis," *European Journal of Obstetrics & Gynecology and Reproductive Biology* 169, no. 2 (2013): 392–96.
2. N. Fritzer and G. Hudelist, "Love is a pain? Quality of sex life after surgical resection of endometriosis: a review," *European Journal of Obstetrics & Gynecology and Reproductive Biology* 209 (2017): 72–76.
3. Georgie Bevan, "Endometriosis: thousands share devastating impact of condition," *BBC News*, October 6, 2019, https://www.bbc.com/news/health-49897873.
4. Carolina Lorençatto, Carlos Alberto Petta, Maria José Navarro, Luis Bahamondes, and Alessandra Matos, "Depression in women with endometriosis with and without chronic pelvic pain," *Acta Obstetricia et Gynecologica Scandinavica* 85, no. 1 (2006): 88–92.

5. Antonio Simone Laganà, Valentina Lucia La Rosa, Agnese Maria Chiara Rapisarda, Gaetano Valenti, Fabrizio Sapia, Benito Chiofalo, Diego Rossetti, Helena Ban Frangež, Eda Vrtačnik Bokal, and Salvatore Giovanni Vitale, "Anxiety and depression in patients with endometriosis: impact and management challenges," *International Journal of Women's Health* 9 (2017): 323–30.
6. Michael J. Sullivan and Joyce L. D'Eon, "Relation between catastrophizing and depression in chronic pain patients," *Journal of Abnormal Psychology* 99, no. 3 (1990): 260–63.
7. Kelly McGonigal, *The Joy of Movement: How Exercise Helps Us Find Happiness, Hope, Connection, and Courage* (New York: Avery, 2019).
8. Marita Lina Sperschneider, Michael P. Hengartner, Alexandra Kohl-Schwartz, Kirsten Geraedts, Martina Rauchfuss, Monika Martina Woelfler, Felix Haeberlin, Stephanie von Orelli, Markus Eberhard, Franziska Maurer, Bruno Imthurn, Patrick Imesch, and Brigitte Leeners, "Does endometriosis affect professional life? A matched case-control study in Switzerland, Germany and Austria," *BMJ Open* 9, no. 1 (2019): e019570.
9. Ibid.
10. Jean A. Gilmour, Annette Huntington, and Helen V. Wilson, "The impact of endometriosis on work and social participation," *International Journal of Nursing Practice* 14, no. 6 (2008): 443–48.

Chapter 5: Week Two: Stress Management

1. Kelly McGonigal, *The Upside of Stress: Why Stress Is Good for You and How to Get Good at It* (New York: Avery, 2016), xxi.
2. Bettina Toth, "Stress, inflammation and endometriosis: are patients stuck between a rock and a hard place?" *Journal of Molecular Medicine* 88, no. 3 (2010): 223–25.
3. Elizabeth A. Stanley, *Widen the Window: Training Your Brain and Body to Thrive during Stress and Recover from Trauma* (New York: Avery, 2019), 29.
4. Kristin Neff, *Self-Compassion: The Proven Power of Being Kind to Yourself* (New York: William Morrow, 2011), 10.
5. Britta K. Hölzel, James Carmody, Mark Vangel, Christina Congleton, Sita M. Yerramsetti, Tim Gard, and Sara W. Lazar, "Mindfulness practice leads to increases in regional brain gray matter density," *Psychiatry Research* 191, no. 1 (2011): 36–43.
6. Cal Newport, *Digital Minimalism: Choosing a Focused Life in a Noisy World* (New York: Portfolio, 2019), 99–109.
7. McGonigal, *The Upside of Stress*, 165.
8. Oliver Hämmig, "Health risks associated with social isolation in general and in young, middle and old age," *PLoS One* 14, no. 7 (2019): e0222124.

Chapter 6: Week Three: Good Food

1. Kelly M. Adams, W. Scott Butsch, and Martin Kohlmeier, "The state of nutrition education at US medical schools," *Journal of Biomedical Education* 4 (2015): 1–7.

2. Fabio Parazzini, Paola Viganò, Massimo Candiani, and Luigi Fedele, "Diet and endometriosis risk: a literature review," *Reproductive Biomedicine Online* 26, no. 4 (2013): 323–36.

3. Agnete Fjerbaek and Ulla B. Knudsen, "Endometriosis, dysmenorrhea and diet—what is the evidence?" *European Journal of Obstetrics, Gynecology, and Reproductive Biology* 132, no. 2 (2007): 140–47.

4. National Institute on Alcohol Abuse and Alcoholism (NIAAA), "Using alcohol to relieve your pain: what are the risks?," https://www.niaaa.nih.gov /publications/brochures-and-fact-sheets/using-alcohol-to-relieve-your-pain.

5. Robin Abcarian, "Column: A few more words on Alzheimer's prevention: Tap water? Caviar? Twinkies?" *Los Angeles Times*, April 6, 2018, accessed March 19, 2020, https://www.latimes.com/local/abcarian/la-me-abcarian-tap-water-20180 405-story.html.

Chapter 7: Week Four: Movement

1. Heba Shaheed, "6 simple exercises to ease endometriosis," medium.com, March 16, 2016, accessed March 14, 2020, https://medium.com/@ThePelvicExpert/6 -simple-exercises-to-ease-endometriosis-a5d2fa3cbd57.

2. Kelly McGonigal, *The Joy of Movement.*

3. Jaclyn P. Maher, Shawna E. Doerksen, Steriani Elavsky, and David E. Conroy, "Daily satisfaction with life is regulated by both physical activity and sedentary behavior," *Journal of Sport and Exercise Psychology* 36, no. 2 (2013): 166–78.

4. Robert J. Gatchel, Randy Neblett, Nancy Kishino, and Christopher T. Ray, "Fear-avoidance beliefs and chronic pain," *Journal of Orthopaedic & Sports Physical Therapy* 46, no. 2 (2016): 38–43.

5. Mike Armour, Justin Sinclair, K. Jane Chalmers, and Caroline A. Smith, "Self-management strategies amongst Australian women with endometriosis: a national online survey," *BMC Complementary and Alternative Medicine* 19, no. 1 (2019): 17.

6. Dayna M. Yorks, Christopher A. Frothingham, and Mark D. Schuenke, "Effects of group fitness classes on stress and quality of life of medical students," *The Journal of the American Osteopathic Association* 117, no. 11 (2017): e17–e25.

Chapter 8: Week Five: Kinder Home + Body

1. Melissa M. Smarr, Kurunthachalam Kannan, and Germaine M. Buck Louis, "Endocrine disrupting chemicals and endometriosis," *Fertility and Sterility* 106, no. 4 (2016): 959–66.

2. Chong-Jing Gao and Kurunthachalam Kannan, "Phthalates, bisphenols, parabens, and triclocarban in feminine hygiene products from the United States and their implications for human exposure," *Environment International* 136 (2020).

3. U.S. Food & Drug Administration, Center for Food Safety and Applied Nutrition, "Parabens in cosmetics," February 4, 2020, accessed August 3, 2020, https://www.fda.gov/cosmetics/cosmetic-ingredients/parabens-cosmetics#are _parabens_safe.

4. United States Environmental Protection Agency, *Glyphosate—Interim Registration Review Decision Case Number 0178*, Docket Number EPA-HQ-OPP-2009-0361, January 2020, www.regulations.gov, Registration Review Decision, EPA, 2020.

Chapter 9: More Tools to Explore

1. Kimberly Y. Z. Forrest and Wendy L. Stuhldreher, "Prevalence and correlates of vitamin D deficiency in US adults," *Nutrition Research* 31, no. 1 (2011): 48–54.
2. Andrew S. Cook, "Lightening your toxic load," in Cook, *The Endometriosis Health & Diet Program* (Toronto: Robert Rose, 2017), 86.
3. Ethan Budd Russo, "Cannabis treatments in obstetrics and gynecology: a historical review," *Journal of Cannabis Therapeutics* 2, nos. 3–4 (2002): 5–35.

Index

About the Author

Jessica Murnane is the founder of Know Your Endo, the author of *One Part Plant*, and a sought-after speaker. She has contributed to or appeared in several magazines and websites including *Bon Appétit, Goop, Shape* magazine, *The Kitchn, mindbodygreen,* and *The Coveteur.* She lives in Charleston, South Carolina, with her family and lots of palm trees.